Thomas Wiltberger Evans

Sanitary Institutions During the Austro-Prussian-Italian Conflict

Conferences of the international societies of relief for wounded soldiers. Anessay

on ambulance wagons. Universal exhibition rewards and letters.

Thomas Wiltberger Evans

Sanitary Institutions During the Austro-Prussian-Italian Conflict
*Conferences of the international societies of relief for wounded soldiers. An essay on
ambulance wagons. Universal exhibition rewards and letters.*

ISBN/EAN: 9783337297343

Printed in Europe, USA, Canada, Australia, Japan

Cover: Foto ©ninafisch / pixelio.de

More available books at **www.hansebooks.com**

SANITARY INSTITUTIONS

DURING THE

AUSTRO-PRUSSIAN-ITALIAN CONFLICT.

CONFERENCES OF THE INTERNATIONAL SOCIETIES OF RELIEF FOR WOUNDED SOLDIERS.

AN ESSAY ON AMBULANCE WAGONS.

UNIVERSAL EXHIBITION REWARDS AND LETTERS.

CATALOGUE OF THE AUTHORS SANITARY COLLECTION.

BY

THOMAS W. EVANS M. D.,

Author of " The United States Sanitary Commission, its origin, history and results.,'
" An Uncles letters to his nephew, on the Constitution of the United States.,''
etc., etc.
Officer of the Legion of Honor.,
Surgeon Dentist to the Emperor Napoléon III
and to the Emperor of Russia.,
United States Commissioner to the Universal Exhibition
Member of the International Jury.

THIRD EDITION.

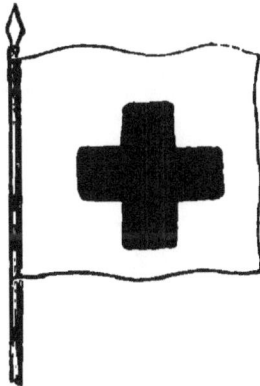

PARIS:

PRINTED BY SIMON RAÇON AND C°.
N° 1, RUE ERFURTH.

1868.

In dedicating to you this book, dear Agnes, I do not propose to give you only a proof of my unalterable affection. I desire also to recognize publicly the part which belongs to you in this work, written with the thought of contributing to the diminution of human suffering.

Was it not you, in fact, who even before our marriage, in the time of our childhood, gave me already at Philadelphia our birth place, the example of an indefatigable charity?

Was it not you, who after our union, for good or for bad fortune, never ceased to assist our fellow creatures, to take care of the sick and to console the afflicted?

Was it not you also, who inspired me with something of your christian charity, and who have constantly aided and approved me, when I have searched the means to render less terrible the sufferings which are caused by war among the human family.

It is therefore with a sentiment of profound gratitude, dear Agnes, that this book is dedicated to you.

THOMAS WILLIAM EVANS.

Bella Rosa, avenue de l'Impératrice, 41.

Paris, 1868.

PREFACE

The work which is now offered to the public has seemed to the writer a proper sequel to *La Commission Sanitaire des États-Unis*, which was published towards the close of the year 1864, and extensively circulated in Europe. The history and example of the United States Sanitary Commission, has exerted a powerful influence upon the organisation and growth of kindred institutions. Old prejudices have been corrected, the practicable and the possible demonstrated, and the friends of humanity and progress everywhere encouraged to new and more vigourous efforts. These were rewarded during the late Austro-Prussian conflict with many splendid results, and have more recently, effected important modifications in the rules of war as practiced among civilised nations.

It was my purpose in the present work to indicate these efforts and results, to show, so far as possible, the actual condition of the recent movements in favor of ameliorating the miseries of war. · No time seemed more favorable to such an undertaking, than when the Great Exposition had assembled at Paris, whatever was most remarkable in connection with modern civilisation, and was offering as it were a new starting-point for every progressive enterprise.

The volume, under the title of *Les institutions sanitaires pendant le conflit Austro-Prussien-Italien*, was published in May last.

The reception which it at once met with was most gratifying, and in again giving it to the public, I am but yielding to the advice of many friends, who see in an English version the means of a wider and more general circulation.

With reference to the execution of the work, I must claim the generous indulgence of the reader.   Many of my notes, as well as the volume itself, were originally written in French, a circumstance which must explain certain faults which could not be avoided without entirely rewriting the book, which in view of my extensive professional and general engagements has been impossible.

A few new facts have been added to the French edition, both in the body of the book and in the appendix.

I most sincerely trust that in its new form, the volume may serve to make better known how much has been done in every part of the world to popularise a great public charity, while not the least among the many pleasant thoughts which it may always suggest in my own heart, will be the remembrance, that while it was my privilege to first repeat in Europe the eventful story of the United States Sanitary Commission, to me also has it been permitted, to signalise to my countrymen and countrywomen, how large and universal has become the interest awakened by that memorable record of patriotism, unselfish devotion, and Christian humanity.

THOMAS WILLIAM EVANS, M. D.

Paris, 1868.

SANITARY INSTITUTIONS

THE AUSTRO-PRUSSIAN-ITALIAN CONFLICT

CHAPTER FIRST

THE SANITARY COMMISSION OF THE UNITED STATES AND THE CONVENTION OF GENEVA

Disposition of modern nations to mitigate sufferings occasioned by war. — Sanitary Commission of the United States. — Initiative of American women. — Conferences of Geneva. — Principles of the Geneva Convention analogous to those expressed in the statutes of American Sanitary Commission. — Establishment of international relief societies favored by several sovereigns.

One of the most touching and at the same time consoling characteristics, which can present itself to the consideration of anyone observing with attention the evils occasioned by war among nations, is the faculty huma-

nity possesses of gathering useful instruction from the very misfortunes that strike
it, the marvellous intelligence exhibited
by people afflicted with war, to invent
measures, for mitigating incalculable sufferings and for opposing boundaries to the
power of the scourge.

A memorable example of the kind was
offered us in the United States, during the
great civil war, which came so unexpectedly
to desolate that prosperous country.

From the outset of this struggle which was
to assume gigantic proportions, a generous
impulse thrilled the heart of the nation; a
grand and sublime thought shone forth in
every soul; since it is a question of war to
the dire extremity, said the people, let us
render it less horrible by surrounding with
our attentions and our solicitude, those who
fight to sustain the rights of the nation. Such

was the sentiment which animated every loyal heart; to the American women however redounds the honor of having given the first impulse to this magnificent popular movement, resulting in the organisation of the Sanitary Commission of the United States, a commission which has rendered inappreciable services to the country, and which we consider one of the greatest blessings the sentiment of charity and humanity has ever given birth to.

Although, in a preceding work, I have related the history and explained the organization of this institution, I may be permitted to retrace here in a few lines its origin and results. I deem it the more useful to recall them briefly to the recollection of the reader, since the American Sanitary Commission has been in reality the type or form upon which are modelled, in a manner more or less faithful, similar societies subsequently created in Europe, particularly the sanitary institutions organized in Germany during the late Austro-Prussian conflict.

When the rebellion broke out in the United States by the attack on fort Sumpter, and President Lincoln had made his first call for the levying of 75,000 volunteers, so many recruits presented themselves, that great confusion was occasioned in the war department, especially in the Medical Bureau. To provide for the wants of an immense multitude of men recruited indiscriminately, and ignorant of the most elementary rules of discipline, would have been a difficult task even for experienced officers; what then must have been the inextricable embarrassment of employees, unacquainted with the means to be employed for procuring indispensable provisions! As for the surgeons, the most

zealous and provident, were often precisely
those who increased the difficulties, and
caused most perplexity to the Medical Bureau, because they were not furnished with
the instruments and supplies which they demanded with importunity.

It was in the midst of this general confusion that associations were formed over all
the vast territory of the Union : in the cities
and even the most remote villages, meetings
were held, inquiries instigated, and mutual
information exchanged, upon the manner of
preparing lint, bandages, and other objects,
necessary for nursing the wounded.

Still these were, to a great extent, isola-
ted aspirations, local efforts, assemblies
which did not act in concert. It was soon
understood that if these efforts of the nation
were to produce expected and desirable fruits,
it was necessary to create a central office,

charged with the duty and responsibility of collecting the offerings, and of distributing them judiciously at the moment and at the place, where they would be the most useful, directing attention to whatever defects might exist in the sanitary service, while at the same time offering the concurrence of a national charity to the Medical Bureau.

On the 25th of April 1861, at the very beginning of the war, about a hundred ladies, belonging to the most distinguished families, assembled at New-York, for the purpose of ascertaining the best means for the realisation of this thought. They drew up a paper addressed to their fellow-towns-women; and appealing afterwards to all their compatriots, interested in their undertaking a number of the most distinguished men of the country, among whom were some of the most celebrated physicians and surgeons.

Through the persistent efforts of these noble women, and the energy of these men of courage and action, all obstacles were finally overcome, the work was realized, the United States Sanitary Commission organized, and the Medical Bureau itself, abandoning the beaten path of routine, united its efforts with those of the Sanitary Commission.

From that moment this institution, without precedent in the history of any people, did not cease to propagate its benefits throughout the land ; and during the long struggle which strewed the country's soil with innumerable victims, every voice united in blessing a work whose benevolent action was felt wherever a soldier suffered, or wherever the blood of a combatant flowed.

To resume in a word, the results obtained by the Sanitary Commission of the United States, I will state that it is known at this

time to have distributed relief representing a
sum of the pecuniary value of one hundred
and twenty five millions of francs ; while it
has probably preserved for the service of the
United States, an army of more than one
hundred thousand men, by its attentions,
rendered to the sick and wounded.

A work so powerful, so fruitful in happy
results, could not fail to attract the attention
of other people, and to interest all those who
are affected by the thought of human sufferings; hence it was that when I had published my book upon the origin and results
of the Sanitary Commission of the United
States, I received from all parts of Europe tes-
timonials of the warmest sympathy for this institution, and several sovereigns, more quali-
fied than private individuals to propagate, and
especially to realize the idea of an analogous
work in Europe, conveyed to the author assu-

rances of the admiration which they entertained respecting the nation, that had known
how to bring to a happy issue an enterprise
as grand as it was original.

In 1863, at the very time when the Sanitary Commission, after having surmounted
every obstacle, was developing itself in all
its force and vigor, an international conference assembled at Geneva, to deliberate upon
the means for establishing a sanitary organization, which should mitigate the horrors of
war and prevent for the future the recurrence
of those heartrending scenes which characterized the battle field of Solferino, scenes
which no one can forget, who witnessed them,
and which, at the time of these deliberations,
were still fresh in the memory of every friend
of humanity.

In the discussions which took place during this memorable meeting, several mem-

bers of the conference expressed the opinion
that a sanitary organization based upon individual initiative, or the spontaneous efforts
of the people was an impracticable chimera.
The reader, who now knows to what prodi-
gious results the American Commission had
arrived at that period, will understand my
astonishment on becoming acquainted with
the debates of the conference. Was it not
indeed strange that such opinions should be
asserted when a glance upon what was passing on the other side of the Ocean, might
have convinced any one of the marvellous
power which lies in the free and spontaneous
action of individuals? Nevertheless, certain
members of the conference did finally call
attention to the Sanitary Commission of the
United States; in short, the project which
emanated from the deliberations of the conference, rested upon principles and senti-

ments similar to those that had given birth to the American institution. In fact, it must not be forgotten that several articles of the Geneva convention of 1864, though expressed in other terms, are found in the statutes of the American association, and that, if the Genevese convention stipulates that wounded soldiers shall be collected and cared for regardless of their nationality, the Sanitary Commission of the United States had acted upon the same principle, by distributing indiscriminately its resources to friends and enemies lying side by side on the bed of suffering. The recognition of the neutrality of all hospital corps, admitted by the Geneva convention, is a reform prolific in results, and which, during the late war in Germany, rendered inestimable services and preserved the lives of thousands of sick and wounded.

I cannot omit remarking that this thought of neutralizing the wounded was entertained, before it was discussed in the Geneva conference, and even before it had been realized by the Sanitary Commission of the United States, as may be seen by the decree which the emperor Napoleon III promulgated during the Italien war, a short time after the victory of Montebello.

This memorable fact is related by the *Moniteur* of the 29th of May 1859, in the following terms :

" The emperor Napoleon III, wishing to diminish, as much as is in his power, the evils occasioned by war, and to give the example for the suppression of unnecessary rigors, has decided, May 28th, that all wounded prisoners shall be delivered to the enemy, without exchange, so soon as their condition may permit them to return to their country."

The spirit of this decree is, we see, entirely conformable to the principles which were subsequently accepted in America and in Europe. However, before exposing the application which these principles have found in Europe, and especially in Germany, we wish to speak of the noble part taken by the women every where, in the work of sanitary reform. I have already mentioned with what spirit of charity and devotion, the American women, consecrated themselves to the sanitary work, and with what perseverance they conducted their admirable enterprise to a happy end. Does not this work which, humble at its beginning, stretched little by little its branches over a large portion of the new world, to extend them afterwards over the whole of Europe, recall to mind the mustard seed spoken of by the scripture, which, humble at its beginning, became a tree under whose shadow suffering humanity reposed !

In Europe as in the new world, the thought of a sanitary reform, destined to bring relief to the wounded and to render less cruel the inevitable sufferings produced by war, has inspired acts of devotion, not only in men who, by their fortune or position, were able to act efficaciously, but has especially animated the women with a noble and holy ardor. Among them many princesses and more than one sovereign have distinguished themselves by the abnegation, zeal and intelligence which they have placed in the service of the humane work to which they dedicated their time and energy. It may be said, I think, that if the reform proposed by the Geneva conference has been welcomed

and immediately put in practice by a large
number of European powers, it was due particularly to the happy influence of a number
of female sovereigns. They knew how to inspire those who surrounded them with something of the spirit of charity that animated
them, and of the ardent sympathy they felt for
the projected work. We know that the Empress of the French was peculiarly favorable
to this sanitary reform; indeed it could not
be otherwise with a princess who, during
her whole career, and even before she wore
an imperial crown, has ever been ready to
alleviate, by personal attentions, the sufferings of the sick and needy. As evidence of
this fact, I could cite several examples, but
it would be superflous; for have we not seen
in these past few years, this sovereign, founding asylums, visiting the hospitals in the
very midst of epidemics, reviving and chee-

ring the sick, and thus meriting the name of sister of charity (*sœur grise*) which the people have given her [1]?

Another great European power had signed the Geneva convention at the same time with France : it was Prussia; here too it was the Queen who came forward, and placing herself at the head of the sanitary movement, with a zeal as persevering as it was admirable, insured its triumph over every obstacle. I shall show in the following pages the part taken by this sovereign in the hospital reforms of the kingdom, and the reader will have an opportunity of appreciating with what intelligent activity, and inexhaustible goodness she inaugurated and consolidated the sanitary organization in Prussia, which has rendered and still renders such great services to that country.

[1] Since writing the above I am permitted to make public an interesting letter written by the Empress, in the Spring of 1862. See Appendix, page 195.

CHAPTER II

Sympathy of the King and Queen of Prussia for the work of the Sanitary Commission of the United States. — Autograph letter from the King. — Groups of voluntary hospital attendants at the different railway stations. — First appearance of the Prussian relief society. — Its activity during the Schleswig-Holstein campaign. — Sending of commissioners to Schleswig.

When war broke out in Germany, my attention was directed naturally, and in a manner quite special, to the hospital and sanitary organizations of that country. It appeared to me that by studying these organizations in belligerent countries, and comparing them with similar institutions which I had investigated in America and elsewhere, some useful information might

be obtained. By repairing to the theatre
of events in order to better examine the
questions which had occured to me, I
considered that I was fulfilling a duty, the
more so because, before the war, their Ma-
jesties the King and Queen of Prussia, had
repeatedly expressed to me their unqualified
sympathy with the work accomplished by
the United States Sanitary Commission, and
had deigned to encourage me in the efforts
I was making to propagate in Europe the
idea of a sanitary enterprise, similar to that
which in America had rendered so great
services to humanity. The following is the
manner in which the King expresses himself
in an autograph letter :

To Mr Thomas W. Evans M. D.

" Accept the assurance of the great interest
derived from the work which you have trans-

mitted me through the agency of the Queen.
She has conveyed to you in my name the
token of esteem which I destined for you on
account of your important medical researches; but I wish, by these lines, to state
the purpose which honors them : the alleviation of suffering in general, and the amelioration of the sanitary condition of armies. "

" WILLIAM.

" Baden, this 13*th* October 1865. "

Would the principles adopted by the Genevese convention answer general expecta-
tion, now that they were put in practice
upon a vast scale? How were the relief
committees going to operate? Will they have
adopted some of the measures tried and
found good during the great war in the

United States? And if they have profited
by the experience of the United States, what
improvements or modifications will they
have introduced in the American work, to
adapt it to the customs of Europe and to the
exigences of a war undertaken under different circumstances? Such were the questions which presented themselves to my
consideration; such was the problem I proposed to investigate.

One of the first things that struck me
when I had entered upon the territory
where important events were being unfol-
ded, was the presence of large numbers of
volunteer hospital attendants at most of the
railway stations. They wore upon the arm
the badge of the international society; the
red cross upon a white ground. They were
there awaiting each convoy, and ready
to render assistance to whatever woun-

ded soldiers, friends or enemies, the train might bring. I was reminded of the volunteer hospital attendants of the American Sanitary Commission, who also prepared at the stations " Refreshment Rooms, " and " Homes, " for the sick and wounded, returned from the fields of battle. But while recognizing with an unfeigned satisfaction the similarity existing between the two organizations, I remarked immediately a difference which seemed to me important. In America female attendants were seen everywhere even at the railway stations, rivalling in devotion the men, while here, there were none. This deficiency struck me, and more than once in the course of this work, I shall have occasion to speak of the absence, regrettable according to our ideas, of women in the hospital service of Germany. But before communicating the reflections which, the operation of the new hospital and sanitary institutions in Germany may suggest, it is advisable perhaps to offer a few explanations, of the manner in which they have originated in that country and particularly in Prussia.

It is known that this power was one of the first to sign the Geneva convention; it was also destined to inaugurate the reform and make the first practical experience of it. Although the King of Prussia signed the treaty on the 24th of August 1864, as early as the month of February of the same year, a relief society had been formed at Berlin; — the Central Prussian Society, — which entered into active service the following month, — the campaign of Schleswig-Holstein having commenced. This campaign, undertaken during the winter, had brought forth sufferings that forcibly invoked public attention. The Central Prussian Society, whose headquarters were at Berlin, made an appeal to the people, and in a few days had at its disposition four thousand thalers. This certainly was not a very considerable sum, nevertheless the committee were prepared to make such a judicious use of it that, from the commencement, the army felt the beneficent action of the institution; and shortly afterwards contributions in kind were received in sufficient abundance, to relieve effectively the most urgent necessities. This committee found itself at the head of an institution without precedent in the military annals of Europe ; consequently it became necessary for it to advance prudently and, if I may so speak, gropingly. It commenced by sending to the theatre of war one of its most distinguished members, Doctor Gurlt, professor in the faculty of

Berlin. This delegate had more particularly
for his mission the studying of the ways and
means for transporting the wounded from
the field of battle. It was not long however
before it was discovered, that it was indis-
pensible for the society to be represented in
a permanent manner upon the field of operations. For this purpose Colonel de Malo-
chowski and Major de Witje, were sent as
delegates of the committee, and, through
the devoted activity of these intelligent men,
a depot was immediately organized in the
city of Flensburg, the very center of military operations, so that lint, instruments of
surgery, bedding, medicines, and alimentary supplies, could be delivered to the
physicians of the army instantaneously and
as they required them.

Although the number of wounded did not
exceed the foresight of professional men,

yet the military hospitals contained more sick and wounded than the space which they could dispose of admitted, and considerable mortality followed. In presence of this fact, the relief society appealed to all the rural proprietors of Schleswig-Holstein, to ascertain if they would be disposed to receive at their homes wounded soldiers. To this appeal the population responded with such eagerness that it was impossible for the society to accept all the offers made. From that moment over crouding ceased in the hospitals, wounds healed more regularly, and the proportional rate of mortality decreased considerably. In addition, the central committee, with resources still restricted, found the means of delivering sums of from twenty to one hundred francs to most of the invalids who left the hospitals.

Such were the acts which the Prussian
Sanitary Commission was able to accomplish during the Schleswig-Holstein war.
We do not see in this, it is true, brilliant
and unexpected results like those which
signalized the beginning of the United States
Sanitary Commission, still it would be un-
just to disparage the spirit which the people
exhibited, from the commencement, in a
work for which they were not prepared.
The central committee of Berlin accomplished, in a sphere restricted in appearance, a very great and very considerable
work in view of the resources possessed,
and the novelty of the enterprise which it
was inaugurating before attentive Europe.
I purposely say that Europe was attentive,
for we must not forget that at the time
when the central committee entered upon its
work, the statutes of the Geneva conference

were still untried, and the realization of the principles which they enunciated appeared scarcely probable, if not impossible to some of the persons who had assisted at the debates of the Conference. Consequently great interest was attached to the enterprise attempted by the Prussian Relief Society; and the happy results obtained have strongly contributed to the general adoption of the international treaty which was signed in the city of Geneva.

After the Schleswig compaign, the central society, faithful to an article of that treaty, remained in active service with the view of preparing during peace the means of succoring the wounded, should war again break out.

CHAPTER III

TRANSFORMATION OF THE CENTRAL SOCIETY INTO AN
INTERNATIONAL RELIEF SOCIETY

Resources of War Departement, however considerable, are generally
insufficient. — Necessity of spontaneous action on the part of po
pulations.—The Prussian Society of Relief to the sick and wounded
obtains the privilege of corporation. — Appeal of the central committee to the nation. — Central depot of Berlin — Reflections
suggested by it to the author. — Statutes of the Prussian Relief
society.

It has been seen in the preceding pages
that, during the campaign of Schleswig-
Holstein, the hospitals were encumbered,
and the surgeons obliged to make great
efforts to render assistance wherever their
presence was required; and yet one would
have supposed that it would have been
otherwise, since not only were there

no great battles fought, during this war, but the organization of the medical service of the Prussian army, particularly its hospital organization, is one of the most complete in existence. Indeed every corps of the Prussian army is amply provided with the material and persons, necessary for the service of three field hospitals and three ambulances (*leichte und schwere Feldlazarethe*). Independently of the Medical corps and a considerable number of nurses, there are sanitary companies in each body of the army; that is to say, detachments of troops specially detailed to take up the wounded and transport them to the ambulances or temporary hospitals.

But however numerous may be the hospital employees, and however perfect the organization of the medical service of an army, there will always be, in the course of a campaign, moments when these employees and this organization will be found insufficient. It is, in truth, absolutely beyond the power of the official administration to provide, on the spot and immediately, for the necessities created by a bloody battle, when many thousands of wounded are demanding succor, as I have lately seen. Where to find in this trying moment surgeons in sufficient number, where to find bandages and lint to dress so many wounds, where to find nurses to attend to so many victims, and when the hospitals are filled with wounded and the supplies of the Medical corps have been consumed, as sometimes arrives in a few days, how, in these moments when the country is exhausted, the population hostile, and communications difficult, how to find medicines, bedding, food and apparatus, are questions which constantly arise and difficulties

which often present themselves. These obstacles may be removed, for it is in these decisive moments that the sanitary institutions
which constitute the subject of our work,
intervene efficaciously, it is then that they
offer their co-operation to the Medical corps
of the army, that they send forward their volunteer nurses, distribute their supplies, and
share the invaluable treasures confided to them
by the people. Thus it was, that the services
rendered by the Prussian Sanitary Society
were appreciated by the war department to
such an extent, that after the Schleswig-Holstein campaign, and in time of peace, the
government not only resolved to protect this
institution, but to give it a greater development. As early as the month of April 1865,
the Central committee was advised that the
King and Queen took the work under their
immediate protection. This determination

was announced to the committee in the following terms :

" Upon a proposition which has been presented to us the 12th of this month, we have
resolved to place under our special protection
the Prussian Society, founded with the view
of succoring, in time of war, sick and wounded soldiers ; we give our protection to this
Society in consideration of the elevated and
important aim it pursues.

    " *Signed :* WILLIAM AND AUGUSTA.

" Berlin, 15*th* April 1865. "

After the war with Denmark, the funds at
the disposition of the central committee were
nearly exhausted; yet new contributions were
made, and on the 1st of January 1866, a
short while before the Society was transformed and entered upon a new sphere of acti-

vity, the condition of its resources presented
the following :

RECEIPTS:

RECEIPTS.	SPECIE.			STOCKS.
	Thl.	Sgr.	Pfg.	Thl.
1. Assets, according to proceding inventory.	261	05	10	5,500
2. Annual contributions. . . .	1,261	—	—	
3. Contributions of local socie- ties.	2,442	21	02	
4. Offerings.	927	13	07	
Divers receipts :				
5. Product of the sale of 2 gold weddings rings. . . .	5	20	—	
6. Product of the sale of dif- ferent stocks..	5,855	24	—	
7. Product of capital placed at interest.	438	—	—	
TOTAL RECEIPTS.	11,197	27	07	

Among the expenditures of this year of
peace, 1865 to 1866, we remark with satisfaction that the largest, about 6,000 francs,
was consecrated to assistance given in specie
to the wounded and invalids of the Holstein
campaign. To sum up the financial condition

of the Prussian Society of relief to the wounded, when war was about breaking out with Austria, it possessed :

In specie, about.	₰ 1,400
In different stocks.	₰ 8,000
TOTAL.	₰ 9,400

It was in the month of April 1866. Already the political horizon was darkening with storm clouds, and minds accustomed to sounding the future, foresaw the possibility of a conflict with Austria. At this time the Prussian Society received from the King the right of corporation. This was a great privilege accorded, for, from the moment it was recognized as a corporation by the State, its individuality was established, and it possessed thereafter the power of selling and buying, of building and endowing, of pleading and defending.

At the same time the Government made known that it would be desirable for the Central committee, whose head-quarters were at Berlin, to become for the future the central organ of public charity, in order to avoid the conflict and confusion which had marked the first efforts of the society at the commencement of the Schleswig campaign. After different communications with the government, and especially after the proclamation in which King William called all Prussia under arms, the central committee modified its statutes and addressed to the nation an energetic appeal, from which we quote a few passages.

" Our king has told us, that faithful to his duty, he has called to arms all his people.

These words of our king exhort us to exert an incessant activity, and to assemble during the days of peace which we still have, all our resources, so that if war breaks out we may be ready, with the blessing of God, to help our brothers, sons, relations and friends, who will go forth to defend the country. "

A few weeks later, the central committee added : " The army is under arms, the moment has arrived when we must put the principles of the Geneva convention in practice. To attain this end we rely upon the devoted cooperation of the entire nation. "

This cooperation was not wanting to the central committee. On all sides local relief societies were organized, which attached themselves to the mother society; and gifts in money and kind were sent forward to Berlin from all parts of the monarchy. When I visited the Prussian Capital, — the war was then at its height, — the central depot of this institution was established in one of the most opulent quarters of the city; but the premises appeared to me a great deal too limited for the use to which they were destined. Offerings had arrived there in abundance, enormous boxes obstructed the passages, objects of every nature, mattresses, oilcloths, instruments, bandages, etc., etc., were laying about without order on the stairways. In the same room persons were busy in receiving the supplies which arrived and in shipping others to the theatre of war; the workmen who packed, labored side by side with those who were unpacking. They were nailing and shouting, the noise of the hammers mingled with the voices of superior employers, who were replying to the comers and goers; orders and demands were addressed on all sides, and at times even violent discussions arose.

All that reminded us of the confusion and tumult which reigned during a few weeks in the medical department at Washington, at the beginning of the civil war. While contemplating the noisy and somewhat confused scene, which presented itself to me at the central depot of Berlin, I could not dispel a sentiment of sadness, in thinking how easy it was in the midst of such a tumult, for an order to be misunderstood, or an urgent expedition retarded. For in like occurences, does not the least delay, or the least error, compromise hundreds if not thousands of existences? I hasten to add, however, that my apprehensions were not founded, and that after having seen closely the difficulties in detail, against which the central committee had to contend, I have been only the better able to appreciate the great things it accomplished, and to recognize with what promptitude, with what order and precision, it distributed the treasures of which it was the depositary. It is proper also to remark that, to enlighten it upon the needs of the army, and to aid it in producing the greatest amount of possible good, the central committee had at its side an essential organ; indeed, as soon as it was realized that war was inevitable, the central committee put itself in correspondence with Count de Stollberg, whom the Government had just named commissary general and inspector of the volunteer hospital service of the Prussian army. The government had made a happy choice in appointing to this post the Count de Stollberg, whose devotion to the sanitary work was well known. He became in this manner the medium between the relief society and the medical bureau of the army, and through his solicitude and vigilance, the committee was always made acquainted with the movements of the troops, and its attention always directed in good time to the points where assistance was urgent.

The organization of the Prussian Relief society seems to me excellent, and as its statutes may be usefully consulted whereever similar institutions are organized, I deem it my duty to reproduce here entirely this useful document.

Statutes of the Prussian society of relief to wounded soldiers.

§ 1.

The Prussian society of relief to soldiers sick or wounded in campaign, has for object :

1st In time of war, to aid the royal administration of ambulances and hospitals, in providing for sick and wounded soldiers ;

2d In time of peace, to prepare suitable means for the accomplishment of this object.

The society must accordingly, in time of

peace, do all in its power to prepare and perfect the asylums destined to receive the sick and wounded during war; it must also interest itself in securing the services of the persons required, and in procuring the necessary materials. In time of war it shall place at the disposition of the military sanitary authorities, its forces and resources.

The society bases its action and relations, with analogous societies of other countries, upon the Geneva convention, of the month of October 1863, and particularly upon the international treaty, of the 4th of January 1864, signed by the king on the 22nd of August 1864.

The society has for motto :

Militi pro rege et patria vulnerato.

§ 2.

The central committee has its head-quarters at Berlin. Provincial and parish societies will be formed : considered as subdivisions of the Prussian society, they will be reunited in a single vast corporation.

The central committee maintains constant and regular correspondence with the provincial and parish societies.

As soon as, in any province whatever of the monarchy, a provincial society shall have been organized and provided with regular statutes, tbe members of the old Central Society, sitting at Berlin, who belong to the said province, will become members of the society of the province where they reside.

The old Central Society which operated at Berlin, will form hereafter, a provincia

society, that of the province of Brandebourg,
and will represent at the same time the local
society of Berlin.

§ 3.

The supreme direction of the corporation
is intrusted to a central committee, charged
at the same time with representing the Prussian society abroad.

The committee is composed of at least 24
members. Fifteen of these members must
reside at Berlin.

The government appoints three commissioners to the central committee, who have for
mission, to aid the committee by their coun-
sels, to serve as mediums between the society
and the war department, in order that the
committee may distribute its succors according to the wants of the army, and connect

its hospital and sanitary service, with that of the ambulances and hospitals of the army. The commissioners of the government, are considered members of the committee and take part therein.

The provincial committee of each of the provincial societies, has the right to send one of its members as deputy to the sessions of the central committee, and each of these deputies of the provinces has a voice in the deliberation of the central committee.

§ 4.

The central committee chooses among its own members, its president and two vice-presidents; a secretary and vice-secretary, and lastly its treasurer. The president convokes the committee; and the committee is under obligation to assemble each time that three of its members shall make the demand for it. The decisions of the committee are determined by a majority of voices; in case of an equal division the voice of the president decides on the vote.

§ 5.

The central committee is charged to hold conferences with the authorities, whenever the interest of the society requires it.

It is authorized :

To look after, in the name and in the interest of the society, business of all kinds; particularly :

To make arrangement and pass contracts ;

To cede and abandon rights and privileges belonging to the society ;

To give receipts ;

To begin suits ;

To name and accept arbitrators ;

To take oath ;

To give power of attorney.

All which the committee will have done in the name of the corporation will be obligatory for the latter. All documents emanating from the committee, must be signed by the president and two members of the committee.

§ 6.

Among affairs also within the province of the committee are :

1. The international relations of the Society with foreign societies and governments;

2. The arrangements to be taken in concert with the Prussian authorities on the subject of the operation of the Society;

3. All which concerns the organization of the Society;

4. The convocation and direction of general assemblies ;

5. Making out the balance sheet of the Society ;

6. The deliberations and resolutions on the subject of the employment of the funds in time of peace ;

7. The urgent measures to be taken at the commencement of war and during its prevalence.

8. The general administration of the Society's funds ;

9. The measures to be taken for augmenting the resources of the corporation ;

10. The correspondance with the provincial and parish societies, unless the statutes of the provincial society specify that the Central committee must correspond directly only with the provincial committee and not with the local or parish societies.

The members of the Central committee were elected among the most respected and esteemed men of the monarchy; they were : Prince de Reuss, président; Messrs Abeken; Count d'Arnim Boytzenbourg, formerly Minister of State, vice-presidents ; Bleichroeder, counsellor to the Minister of Commerce; Caspar, counsellor at the Court of Appeals ; de Decker, court printer; Lieutenant general de Derenthall; Professor Firmenich-Richart : de Gruner, Doctor de Langenbeck, Doctor Gurlt, etc., etc.

CHAPTER IV

COMBAT OF LANGENSALZA

Obstinacy of the struggle. — The town of Langensalza encumbered with wounded. — Complete insufficiency of resources in the medical service of the Hanoverian army and the Prussian detachment. — Distress of the surgeons. — Their joy at the sight of the relief sent forward by the central committee of Berlin.

Hardly had war been inaugurated before the central committee of the Prussian society had the opportunity of demonstrating to all, how powerful was the organization created by the corporation, and with what favor its appeal to patriotic and humane sentiments, had been received by the entire nation.

On the 28th June, a detachment of Prussian troops, about five thousand strong,

and almost all natives of Berlin, had marched
to meet the Hanoverian army, which was moving towards the South in order to effect a
junction with the Bavarian troops. The shock
between the Prussian corps and the main body
of the Hanoverians was very violent; both
sides fought with extreme obstinacy, and the
contest lasted for five hours. The Prussians,
after displaying prodigies of valour, were
obliged to fall back, which they did in good
order. The Hanoverian army experienced
enormous losses; and the day, although glorious for the flag of Hanover, proved clearly
the inutility of a prolonged struggle against the
Prussian forces. The Hanoverians retired upon
the town of Langensalza, and the Prussians
camped in the neighborhood. The bloody
combat was not yet terminated, when the insufficiency of resources which the Prussian
medical Corps could dispose of, was felt in a

cruel manner; and as to the resources of the Hanoverians, they were nearly nothing, as we are going to show.

Such was the situation when the royal commissioner to the central committee of the Prussian Relief Society, Count de Stollberg, received information at about 5 o'clock in the afternoon, that there were fifteen hundred wounded at Langensalza, who were absolutely in want of bread. Immediately, the central committee, with a most commendable activity, responded to the call; after midnight, three special convoys left the Berlin station, bearing the succors of the Sanitary Society upon the field of battle. Among the supplies sent forward, were 1072 bandages, representing all together a length of 8125 yards of linen ; 150 plaster preparations, 4 bottles of chloroform, 124 mattresses, 150 compresses, 500 shirts, 102 towels, 100 pairs of socks, lint, slippers, wadding, drawers, surgical instruments, chocolate, and a host of other things destined to relieve or revive the wounded. We see that the committee had shown itself provident and was ready at the first appeal to fulfil its duty nobly and worthily.

One of its members accompanied the expedition, as also eight physicians, and several male and female volunteer nurses, among whom were six deaconesses of the Institution of Protestant Sisters. At Magdebourg several other physicians and nurses united themselves with the members of the Relief Society. The central committee had taken care to telegraph to the local committee of Gotha, the order to prepare vehicles for receiving the supplies shipped, so that no delay was encountered and the convoy reached the little town of Langensalza early in the morning. Here was a sad spectacle. Langensalza was still occupied by the Hanoverians, and although a considerable part of their wounded had already been removed out of the town, there still remained more than a thousand of them, and about three hundred Prussians, distributed in fifteen different quarters. The Hanoverian surgeons were endeavoring to make up by their zeal, for their insufficiency in number; under the skilful direction of their chief, Doctor Stromeyer, one of the most eminent German military surgeons, they accomplished prodigies of devotion, but they were in want of everything which could have rendered such efforts useful.

Neither were the Prussian surgeons in sufficient number to give necessary attentions to such a multitude of wounded. Indeed no one was prepared for so terrible a carnage; the hospital service was wanting not only in nurses, but, strange to say, it did not even possess the necessary material for arranging a single ambulance hospital; so the wounded Hanoverians and Prussians were placed upon such straw as could be hastily procured; some were laying upon the ground; few were they to whom a bed, furnished with a straw matting, had been given. The army surgeons, exhausted by fatigue, were distressed at the sight of so much suffering which they were powerless to alleviate. We may judge then of the satisfaction experienced, when they saw the arrival of a long train of wagons which brought them all those different things so much needed: bedding, lint, bandages, compresses, and provisions! We may fancy their gratification when they saw coming to their aid, the male and female nurses and the physicians the Relief Society had sent!

Every thing was soon transformed and a better aspect of affairs followed. All the wounded Prussians and Hanoverians were installed in good beds, order was established and anxieties ceased.

CHAPTER V

THE BATTLE OF SADOWA

Magnitude of the struggle. Heart-rending scenes. — Large numbers
of wounded remain several days without dressing of wounds. —
Activity and devotedness of Prussian physicians. — Ambulances
in the villages surrounding the battle field. — Solicitude and kindness of the surgeons in the field hospitals. — The wounded in
the hospitals of Milowitz and Sadowa.

It has been shown in the preceding chapter, with what intelligence and energy the
central committee of the Prussian Society
gave aid and assistance to the medical
department of the army, at the first conflict between the hostile forces. Yet that,
was so to speak, only the first trial made by
the institution of its forces. From that moment it became conscious of what it could

realize, and when graver and more decisive events occurred to astonish Germany and Europe, almost immediately after the combat of Langensalza, the Prussian Society proved in a splendid manner the great services a work based upon the free cooperation of a united people can render in these solemn moments.

The Prussian troops had penetrated into Bohemia by the narrow defiles of Saxony and Riesengebirge. A series of bloody battles had conducted them to the banks of the Elbe before the fortress of Konigsgraetz. Here upon the hills and in the vast plain which are near that city, the grand and memorable battle took place, which will remain in the annals of history as one of the greatest events of the 19th century.

More than five hundred thousand combatants confronted each other on the mor-

ning of the 3^d of July. The shock was
terrible; from eight o'clock in the morning
until five in the evening, the roar of cannon
was incessant; and when, towards evening,
the King of Prussia, who had directed the
battle, put himself in pursuit of the formi-
dable Austrian army that he had just con-
quered, more than forty thousand wounded
strewed the immense space which stretches
from the village of Sadowa to Chlum, and
from Nechanitz to the fortress of Konigsgraetz. The bloody scene of Solferino,
however cruel and terrible it was, cannot be compared to the immense carnage
which characterized the day of Sadowa.
When the Sanitary companies of the
Prussian army explored the field of battle
an indescribable spectacle was witnessed.
Thousands of Austrians, whole squadrons
of men, were lying upon the soil in the atti-

tude which they had at the moment when,
arrived within reach of the Prussian projec-
tiles, they had fallen overwhelmed by the
deadly fire; in the midst of the dead, innumerable wounded were lying and implo-
ring assistance at the hands of their con-
querors. Among the Prussians the scene
was not less heart-rending. Thousands of
men were laying pell mell upon the ground,
some destroyed by the Austrian squadrons
which had charged with reckless impe-
tuosity; others wounded by the conical
balls of the infantry, or mutilated by the
shot of the artillery, which, placed upon
the heights of Chlum and Nechanitz, had
swept the Prussian ranks. We may easily
fancy the work which the Austrian and
Prussian surgeons had to do on this bloody
day; the Prussian surgeons particularly, for we must remember that the Aus-

trian army in its retreat left almost all its wounded upon the field of battle, abandoning to the generosity of the enemy the task of picking up and providing for them. The surgeons of the Prussian army did not fail in this duty, as will be seen further on; they took care of Prussians and Austrians with an equal solicitude; in acting thus, Prussia was not only obeying a natural sentiment of generosity and humanity, but was fulfilling the engagements to which she had subscribed in signing the treaty of Geneva.

To have fulfilled such engagements conscientiously after this day of carnage, was a glorious work, but one of extreme difficulty. During three days and nights the sanitary companies explored, without intermission, the battle field, taking up the wounded with solicitude and tenderness; yet however car-nest may have been the disposition to carry succour to all indiscriminately, many wounded died before they could be transported to the temporary hospitals. How, indeed, was it possible to organize immediately hospitals in sufficient number to receive so many thousands of wounded? These had been picked up and placed in carts and wagons hastily collected; but where were they to be transported now? A part of these unfortunate beings had to remain in vehicles and endure for a long time unheard of tortures, in spite of the assiduous attentions of the Prussian surgeons, who, worn out with fatigue, sustained themselves by a supreme effort and by the sentiment which they had of the grandeur of their task.

When I arrived upon the field of battle, a little order had commenced to show it self.

Volunteer physicians had arrived from all quarters, and the benevolent influence of the central committee of the Prussian Society began to be sensibly felt. I did not meet a wounded man who had not already received intelligent attention. Besides, if a large number of wounded, had remai· ned in the transport wagons, or upon the battle field two entire days without having their wounds dressed, we must remember that the carnage took place over an immense extent of ground; that many wounded, having sought shelter in the houses abandoned by the countrypeople, had become exhausted there, and that it became necessary to explore villages several leagues distant from each other in order to discover them.

As soon as the first duties were fulfilled, the surgeons organized the hospital service with an admirable precision, and with an appearance of uniformity which left nothing to be desired. Those who were slightly wounded were immediately conducted, some to the neighboring towns of Reichenberg, Horsitz, and Gitshin in Bohemia, and others to Prussia and Saxony. Those who were severely wounded and could not endure the journey, were established in the villages situated on the battle ground; and five days after the fight there was not a village within the circumference of four leagues that was not filled with wounded. I visited with the liveliest solicitude these extemporaneous hospitals, and I can not express the profound impression I felt every time when I saw, at the entrance of one of these hamlets, sadly floating upon the principal house of the place, the white flag, which indicated to the passer by, that there were here, lying

upon beds of suffering, the victims of a
scourge which is said to be indispensable to humanity. Still in each of these
asylums I had occasion also to admire
the admirable devotion of the Prussian surgeons and nurses. They were there, ad-
ministering affectionately to the wants of
those entrusted to their care. In each asy-
lum there were at most, about twenty patients; so the physicians knew them all
by name, questioned them with care,
attached themselves to them, and became
in turn beloved by these unfortunate sufferers. I shall never forget a scene which I
witnessed in the little village of Milowitz.
In a wooden house, composed of a ground
floor or single story, about twenty wounded
were collected in a large room. The hall was
well lighted and the air circulated freely.
On entering this room I was received by

the physician in charge, with that courtesy, to which all the Prussian military surgeons I had met, had accustomed me. He conducted me to a bed where a young Hungarian soldier was lying; a wound received full in the breast was not looking badly, but the leg was swollen. There was evidently a bone fractured near the ankle, and the ball had remained in the wound; still there existed some doubt on this subject. When I arrived in the hospital, the chief of the medical service of the Prussian army, Professor Langenbeck, the celebrated surgeon, had just entered; he went immediately to the wounded young man, near whom were three other physicians. Nothing could be more touching than the solicitude with which the surgeon in chief and the other physicians examined the patient. Mr de Langenbeck, while probing the wound, addressed words full of kindness to the sufferer; he encouraged him to support patiently a pain which he could not spare him. I followed with undisguised admiration the skilful hands of the surgeon, when suddenly turning towards us he said: " The ball is here ". Then addressing himself to the patient he added : " Now be at rest, my boy; you shall soon return home to those who love you. "

This fact is cited not simply to exhibit a trait of goodness and humanity, but because I believe that in a large number of cases, an encouraging word renders less cruel the sufferings of the wounded in foreign countries, far from those who bear them interest and attachment. In hospitals where the sick are nursed by women, they will often find opportunities to speak of the absent country and those they have left there; but in the military hospitals that I visited in the vil-

lages of Bohemia, there were none of these
women by the bedside of the wounded. To
see the gentleness and goodness of the nurses
and physicians, one would say that they wished to assure to their patients the same cares
and attentions that sisters of charity would
have shown for them. An example of this devotion of the surgeons in the Prussian army
is still present in my mind. Count Harrach
possessed in the village of Sadowa a large
sugar refinery. During the battle this establishment, for a moment the center of
a struggle, was riddled with shot. After
the action the manufactory was transformed
into a hospital ; the beds were in the large
work shop on the ground floor, placed against
the walls and the machines, and also in
the upper galeries. All this was organized
with so perfect a knowledge of sanitary principles that, on entering the establishment,

I discovered myself in a spacious hospital, well lighted and provided with an excellent ventilation. Here were placed about fifty wounded, whom a physician and his assistants were attending, with fraternal solicitude. There was among other patients an inhabitant of the place. A few moments before my arrival this man had picked up a bomb, in the court, which he supposed extinguished and the projectile had burst in his arms, and wounded him frightfully. He was lying upon his bed of pain, and death near at hand. But, after all, he had the satisfaction of being surrounded by his wife and children in that trying hour. The surgeon of the establishment who accompanied me said : "Certainly that man is to be pitied, but the young Italian you see yonder, and who is going to die, is still more unfortunate, because he will die far from his friends and his country.

It especially is our duty to mitigate as much as possible, by the affectionate attention we give him, the poignancy of such a death. ''

All these hospitals scattered in the villages of Bohemia, were in communication with each other through the medium of daily reports. Sanitary inspectors visited them frequently, and Mr de Langebenck particularly, indefatigable in the accomplishment of his duty, was continually present in these establishments, to encourage the zeal of the surgeons and to aid them by his knowledge and experience.

CHAPTER VI

Important convoys shipped to the theatre of war. — Depots established in Bohemia and on the banks of the Mein. — International
character of the Prussian Relief Society. — *Buffets* established in
the stations of the railways to distribute refreshments to the
troops. — Prussian society distributes books. — Disinterestedness
and devotedness of the agents of the Society. — The journal
Kriegerheil.

I have stated that, after the first days of
confusion, the wounded of the battle of Sadowa, Austrians as well as Prussians, were
accommodated with good beds and received
all the attention demanded by their condition. I have also said that, from the outset,
the influence of the Prussian Society had
been felt in the hospitals established upon

the field. Indeed to this society redounds in a great measure the merit, of having foreseen the wants that were going to arise, and of having known how to take suitable precautions to provide the medical officers with sufficient means to meet all the requirements of the situation. At the very moment when the first battles took place in the defiles of Saxony and Bohemia, the committee sent forward to these countries a shipment of medical and sanitary supplies having a total weight of more than 50 tons, together with 440 casks of wine. The convoy arrived at Gitschin the day before the battle of Sadowa, and the King of Prussia, after having personally conferred with the members of the committee that followed it, ordered that the materiel should be distributed in the field hospitals, which had been established in the different places where

the Prussians had been victorious, from Na-
chod to the town of Gitschin. A part of the
goods, nevertheless was reserved for the
wounded that were constantly brought back
from the different battle fields. The convoys
of wounded formed a long line of carriages
advancing slowly and with difficulty. When
the delegates of the Society met these wounded a sad sight was offered them : in heavy
wagons, men were lying upon straw, who,
after having received a first dressing of their
wounds, had remained from thirty to forty-
eight hours without food. All the resources
of the country had been exhausted, and one
cannot think without shuddering, of the
fate which had inevitabily befallen a portion
of these men, if the commissioners of the
Relief society had not arrived there, at the
decisive moment, to offer provisions to the
sufferers, and recall them, as it were, to life.

A few days after, a more considerable train started out from Berlin. The battle of Sadowa had been fought, and the Prussian army was moving rapidly upon Vienna. Another battle not less bloody was anticipated, and it was necessary at the same time to face the double exigences of the moment. One of the convoies forwarded by the Society on receiving the news of the great battle, had an approximative value of 60,000 dollars, and among the things composing it, were 4 tons of ice, destined for the service of the hospitals. The committee sent forward every day, during a fortnight, a train of supplies for Bohemia. To introduce order in an enterprise so great and so difficult, the necessity was felt of establishing grand depots upon the very theatre of operations. From these the field hospitals could be aided according to their wants, and relief

carried promptly to the wounded wherec-
ver a serious engagement should demand the
solicitude of the Society's delegates. Such
depots were speedily organized at Turnau,
Gitschin, and especially at Koeniginhof, Trau-
tenau, Brunn, Pardubitz, Wurzbourg, and
Wertheim. But in spite of the precautions and
wise measures, which the central committee
had taken, the supplies destined for the army
of Bohemia experienced often regrettable delays, on account of the encumbrance which
existed on the rail ways. I could not resist a
feeling of sadness at the sight of the numerous
wagons which remained whole days in the
railway stations from Dresden to Prague.
These delays were the more lamentable from
the fact that while considerable shipments
of provisions were spoiling in the stations,
pressing wants were felt in the hospitals of
Brunn and the vicinity, where the cholera

was raging with violence. It would have been easy to have sent the shipments of the Society to Prague, by organizing a transport service on the Elbe; but unfortunately the Saxon commander of the fortress of Koenigstein, a fortress which commanded the river, had declared that he would sink every transport that passed under the guns of the place. This was a deplorable decision in every respect, for it must not be forgotten that the Society of Relief to the wounded was based upon an international principle; and in forbidding it the free navigation of the Elbe, precious succor was withheld not only from the sick and wounded Prussians, but also, and particularly, from the Austrians and Saxons themselves, who were in considerable number in all the hospitals of Bohemia.

At the same time that the society was exerting an incessant activity in assisting the

sick and wounded of the armies that were
operating in Austria, it exhibited a foresight
and solicitude no less great, in regard to the
troops that were acting in Bavaria and upon
the banks of the Mein. Always acquainted in
good time with the movements of the army,
the central committee of the society directed
its shipments, provisions, and nurses, upon
points where engagements were likely to take
place. In this manner sixty convoies were at
different times despatched to those quarters,
so that, through the active and intelligent
intervention of the Relief society, the army
surgeons had at their disposal abundant resources during the bloody days of Kissingen
and Wertheim. What particularly struck me
in the manner of acting of this society, was
that, notwithstanding the enthusiasm exclusively Prussian and patriotic, which animated
every soul at this time, and conducted the

6

SANITARY INSTITUTIONS

Prussians to brilliant successes, it did not abjure an instant its international mission. It distributed its aid impartially to the children of Prussia and to their adversaries. I might simply call to mind the fact that, in the field and regular hospitals, among which the society distributed its supplies, there were always two and even three times as many Austrians as Prussians, but more distinguishing circumstances show to what extent the society was influenced by the sentiment of its international duties. It sent repeatedly, considerable sums of money to the Austrian relief societies, particularly that of Prague.

A large number of volunteers, belonging to the first families of the country, accompanied, without any remuneration, the trains despatched by the society. These volunteers watched over the articles forwarded, and undertook the distribution of the different objects, according to the instructions of the central committee. When the goods could not continue their route on the railway, the agents of the society obtained horses and wagons, and by reason of perseverance arrived in opportune time at the place of destination. For this object, upon the order of the Queen of Prussia, sixty horses and thirty carriages were placed at the disposition of the agents of the society to effect the transportation of materials, sent by the committee of Berlin, from Dresden to Bohemia.

In general, the beneficent action of the Queen was often felt when it became desirable to aid the society in accomplishing its mission in an effective manner. Sometimes this sovereign and the princess royal, came to the bureaux of the society, to encourage by their presence, the ladies occupied in preparing linen and various objects which were to be

82 SANITARY INSTITUTIONS

forwarded to the army; at other times they visited the large towns of the country in order to stimulate the zeal of the local societies. In this way it was, that the shipments from the provincial societies came to be occasionally very considerable.

The states allied to Prussia, also placed at the disposition of the central committee the products of public benevolence. The free city of Bremen for instance, despatched to Berlin at one time, 8,000 dollars in specie, 400 casks and 1,300 bottles of wine, 380 bottles of port, 900 pounds of tobacco, 47,000 cigars, 2,000 pounds of sugar, and 1000 of rice; the days following, shipments as considerable arrived from this same city and the grand duchy of Oldenbourg, while the city of Hamburg sent immense quantities of ice.

The central committee distributed with intelligence and without parsimony the resources it posessed. After the battle of Sadowa, and shortly after the treaty of Nickols-bourg, it made a shipment to Prague which, by its proportions, reminded me of 'those forwarded at times by the United States Sanitary Commission to the federal army. This train or convoy was composed of 22 wagons, and 1 notice among the supplies then sent 50,000 pounds of meat, 34,000 bottles of red wine, 1,500 bottles of cognac, 20,000 pairs of slippers, 5,000 flannel belts, 62,000 cigars and a host of other things as useful as varied.

Independently of the depots where it stored its supplies, the Relief society had organized at the principal railway stations, particularly at the branchline or junction stations, grand *buffets* where its agents were busied in distributing succor to the wounded who were passing, as well as to the field hospitals established in the vicinity of these stations.

Pardubitz, for example, is a railway station on the line leading from Dresden to Vienna and forms a point of junction for several branch roads. From eight to ten thousand men were in garrison there, and towards the end of July the military hospitals of the place were crowded with cholera patients. At this important point the society had established a principal depot which was able to supply the hospitals with every thing necessary for their sick and wounded, and with all the food suitable for convalescents. In addition it had fixed in the railway station one of these *buffets* of which I speak, in order to be better able to distribute its help to the troops that passed, or were temporarily stationed there. It gave daily to each soldier, convalescent or suffering, beef soup, meat, a large glass of wine, a small glass of cognac, with sugar or fresh water, bread, cigars, and, in the morning, a cup of coffee and sweetened bread. From the month of May to July, the number of soldiers passing through Pardu- bitz, and assisted by the society amounted, on an average, to three hundred daily. Another branch of this kind, established at Bodenbach, an important station on the railway from Dresden to Vienna, distributed in the same manner, and in the same time, refreshments to 5,500 convalescents, and to 5,000 well men, fatigued from long travel. This branch establishment, entrusted to the direction of M' Auerbach, a distinguished professor of Ber- lin, who had voluntarily offered his services to the society, this establishment, I say, pla- ced each day 500 rations at the disposal of the troops who passed, and each ration con- sisted of a half pound of meat, a loaf of white bread, a goblet of wine, a small glass of brandy and a glass of sugared water, for the soldier

in health : if the soldier was unwell or convalescent, he was offered another soup
or broth. It is to be regretted that in such
cases, these branch establishments did not
have at their disposition the excellent beef
extract of Borden, which makes one of the
best broths that can be offered to convalescents.

The foresight of the society was not restricted to establishing these grand buffets; in
most of the places which were points of
junction for branch railways, the central
committee had established hospitals destined
to receive sick soldiers arriving at the station and unable to continue their route. These
establishments, provided with everything
necessary for the treatment of the sick, and
conducive to their comfort, rendered important services to the army, particularly
when the cholera came to add its horrors to

those of war. At the same time that the society was in this manner succoring the sick
and wounded upon the very theatre of war,
it also distributed its benefits among those
crowding the large hospitals of Berlin, Breslau, Dresden and most of the principal towns
of Prussia. The directors of these hospitals
and the sick whom I had occasion to question
on the subject, willingly and unanimously
acknowledged the services, for which they
were indebted to the relief society. Always
ingenious in finding an opportunity to fulfil
its mission nobly, by giving every possible
comfort to the sick, it appealed to the booksellers and publishers, to engage them to
furnish, as offerings to the society, such
books as might enable the sick and wounded
to support their sufferings more patiently,
by affording them attractive or profitable
reading. A response to the appeal of the

central committee was made and a large
number of books sent, which were classed
with intelligence. A committee, appointed by
the society, and composed of booksellers
and men of learning , formed very varied
collections of these donations and distributed
them in the field hospitals. as well as those of
Berlin and other cities.

I was particularly struck, while looking
over the list of the various books, with the
happy idea manifested by introducing in these
improvised libraries a very large number of
Italian, Hungarian and Sclavonian works; the
sick and wounded of the Austrian army,
nursed by Prussia, being much more numerous than the Prussian sick, and composed in
part of Italians, Hungarians and Poles, it was
determined that they should profit alike by
the benefits of the measure adopted. This
measure had been taken especially with a

view to the convalescents. Indeed the society proved itself constantly, as interested in aiding them, as it was attentive in lavishing its cares upon the sick. It employed a sum of about 150,000 francs (30,000 dollars) to send convalescent soldiers, officers and surgeons to watering places; and the day the Prussian army entered Berlin, it delivered to every convalescent soldier in the hospitals of that city, regardless of nationality, 8 francs in specie, and two bottles of red wine.

In short, at the end of the war, the Prussian Society of Relief to the wounded, had expended in specie a sum of about two millions of francs, for completing its supplies of provisions, and in relieving the wounded ; on the other hand it had received in kind, and distributed articles of a value estimated at six million francs. Certainly those are con-

siderable sums ; but the intelligent manner
in which these treasures have been distributed, has, so to speak, doubled the value
of them. It is proper to add moreover that, if
the Society has been able to obtain so great
results, it has been especially due to the
energy and self-sacrifice of its agents, who
have fulfilled everywhere, voluntarily and
without remuneration, their noble and difficult mission with a perseverance as admirable as it was unfaltering. In justice also
we must observe, that the Prussian Government seconded powerfully the efforts of the
Society, in authorizing it to use gratuitously
the railways, post and telegraph.

   To place itself in communication with the
public, the Prussian Society of Relief to the
wounded, had founded a special organ, the
Kriegerheil (Soldiers Salute), an organ in
which it gave the public an account of all its

operations, and made frequent appeals to the patriotism and humanity of the Prussian people. This organ continues to appear; it rendered good service during the war and no doubt, now, in time of peace, is still useful in engaging the populations to prepare, during days of tranquility, that which will benefit suffering humanity when the day of trouble arrives.

CHAPTER VII

Services rendered by these orders during the war. — Hospitals of Berlin. Activity of the Queen and Princess Royal of Prussia in favor of the relief societies.

If I have exhibited in the preceding pages the services rendered by the Prussian Society of Relief to the wounded, it is not because it was the only institution of this kind organized by the spontaneous concurrence of the people; I have enlarged upon the results obtained by this society, because it was the one established upon an international principle, and the one possessing also, the most considerable resources. Besides it, there were other relief societies, such as the society of *Kœnig Wilhelm*, and the Society of relief to the army; which had likewise for their mission the succoring of the wounded. Endeavors were made, without success, to effect a coalition between these and the Prussian society; the society *Kœnig Wilhelm*, nevertheless, charged the central committee of Berlin with the distribution of the relief in kind, which it forwarded to the army.

An institution that rendered great services in the hospitals, during the whole war, was the order of the Knights of Saint John. This order, restored in Prussia in **1812**, had until latterly, been only honorary. It is still necessary to be descended from noble parents in order to become a member of it. Already at the time of the Schleswig-Holstein campaign the members of this order, recollecting the elevated mission of the ancient Knights of Saint John, of whom they considered themselves the continuators, wished to be useful by consecrating themselves to nursing the sick and wounded soldiers. During the campaign against Denmark, the order of Saint John had organized a sanitary service, and had sent several of its members to the hospitals and to the battlefield.

When the war broke out between Prussia and Austria, the former government conferred on the grand master of the order of Saint John, Count Stollberg-Wernigerode, the title and powers of commissary general and military inspector of the volunteer hospital service. He was also appointed government commissioner, to the central committee of the Society of Relief to the wounded. This society, through the earnest and cordial concurrence of Count Stollberg, contracted

7

an intimate alliance with the order of
Saint John. A member of the order received
the special mission of maintaining relations
of fraternization between the Society and
the order of Knights. By this union the
Relief Society was enabled to extend its
operations greatly, for every where, upon
the wide field of events the Knights of
the order of Saint John were present
as delegates of their Grand Master. By a
special combination, these Knights were
almost always delegates at the same time
of the Relief Society. It was these Knights
who were most frequently placed at the
head of the numerous depots which the
Society had established in Austria; it was
they who in their quality of hospital volunteers, acquainted the Relief Society with
the wants of the different hospitals in
which they were serving.

The order of Saint John is an evangelical protestant institution. Throughout the
whole war it did not cease to render eminent services; it generously accepted for
its line of conduct the principles of the
international convention of Geneva, and
lavished its attentions without distinction
upon friends and enemies. Since it has
thus been, since it has become, by the
very force of circumstances, the most
important hospital institution of Prussia,
would it not be desirable, to better accomplish the end in view, that it should
not remain purely an aristocratic order,
but on the contrary enlarge its lists by
permitting that every man who should
have distinguished himself by personal
bravery or by services rendered to suffering
humanity, might obtain the honor of being
a Knight of the order, and might bring to

it the cooperation of his experience and
devotion.

Rivaling in zeal the Knights of the order
of Saint John, were the Knights of the catholic order of Malta. Associating themselves in the arduous efforts of the sanitary
companies, the members of these two orders have courageously done their duty
upon the battle fields, and in the field
hospitals, as well as in their quality of
commissioners intrusted with conducting
the trains sent by the Relief Society and
with distributing the supplies forwarded.
I have remarked that the Prussian Relief
Society had not succeeded in centralizing
in its own hands the resources of the
other analogous societies which were in operation at Berlin. It is proper to add however
that there did not exist between these societies any antagonism, and that all carried into

the accomplishment of their task the same earnestness and the same ardor.

Spontaneous offerings, the efforts of public benevolence, are not however limited to relief societies. They are reproduced elsewhere and whenever local circumstances exact a certain independence in the assistance given.

It is thus that in the single city of Berlin, when some ten or more great military ambulances and seven permanent hospitals were in operation, twenty-three private hospitals had been improvised in the space of a few weeks; a large number of families in all the provinces had asked for and adopted either the sick or convalescent, and in addition many landed proprietors had transformed their *chateaux* into hospitals, and had taken convalescents to their homes in order to surround them with kind attentions.

The same devotedness and the same solicitude which we had observed among the Prussian surgeons in the field ambulances, we
again discovered at Berlin in the civil and
military surgeons who had united their
efforts to attend to the thousands of wounded
distributed in all the quarters of the capital.
In general the Berlin hospitals were neatly
kept; but almost always something was wanting in the way of a proper system of ventilation : this serious inconvenience was remarked especially in the great Charity hospital ;
an immense edifice in which a multitude of sick and wounded were collected.
The air did not circulate sufficiently, and to
make it penetrate throughout the building, it
was necessary to open the windows and thus
create currents of air always dangerous in
such circumstances.

A Hospital well aired and lighted, was the

provisional hospital established in the catholic house of the Sisters of Saint-Hedwig. Here at last we found, that, the absence of which had so painfully impressed us in most of the hospital establishments of Prussia, females to nurse the sick. Here, in the house of the Sisters of Saint-Hedwig, we saw the sisters assiduous in attentions to the sick; and the surgeon relieved of great responsibility, knowing that the prescribed dressing would be performed with promptness and gentleness. Indeed, I have assisted at dressings undertaken by these holy women; and avow in all sincerity that, in my opinion, it would have been difficult for even the most expert surgeon to have accomplished them more skillfully and intelligently. There were also in this house reserved rooms, very clean, well aired, and well furnished, where wounded officiers received all the attentions necessitated by their condition. At the time we visited the establishment all the rooms were occupied by Austrian officers wounded at the battle of Sadowa.

I have just said that the absence of female nurses was painfully felt in most of the Prussian hospitals. It must not be understood however, that they were missing there entirely. Far from it : evangelical deaconess, a large number of sisters of Charity and catholic nuns, had been spontaneously directed wherever their holy mission became necessary, and to their eminent services, was joined the cooperation of women of every rank in society, who voluntarily took part in the admirable and arduous task of aiding the physician, to restore to health those whose death seemed inevitable, or to render less painful the last hours of those visited by death. There was in Prussia a woman

who, by her goodness, her intelligence and
position, knew how to cheer the heart of
the faltering and inspire other women of her
country with the noble ardor that animated
herself. This woman was the Queen of Prussia. She did not limit herself to patronizing
the relief societies that were established
in all the provinces of the kingdom, at
Breslau and Magdebourg; but often accompanied by the Princess Royal, she herself visited the sick and wounded; and we shall never forget the emotion experienced when, at
Berlin, having permitted us to accompany
her, we saw her address to the wounded, to
the Austrians as well as to the Prussians,
words of kindness and consolation. The
sick regarded her with admiration and all
without exception blessed her for her goodness.

In short, it must be acknowledged that during the brief period of that great campaign on the Mein and in Bohemia, Prussia made energetic and efficacious efforts to provide for and comfort her sick and wounded soldiers, and has never departed from the international obligations imposed upon her by the Geneva convention.

She has nursed always and everywhere in Bavaria, Saxony and in Austria, her own children and her enemies with the same solicitude. It would be difficult for me to forget the affecting scene I witnessed at Radeberg, a small town in Saxony noted for its mineral waters. A number of Austrian convalescents had arrived there for the purpose of using the waters. They were accompanied by some of the Prussian surgeons who had attended them while in the hospitals. When the time came for bidding farewell to the surgeons, the men, gathering around those to whom

they were indebted for the preservation of life
took their hands and kissed them affectionately and then, by a spontaneous movement
formed a circle around them, and saluted
them three times with the heartiest acclama-
tions.

CHAPTER VII

The Saxon Relief society. — General de Reitzenslein. — Sanitary society of Wurlembourg. — Elevated views of the Queen of Wurtembourg upon the mission of sanitary institutions. — The *Badischer Frauenverein.*. — Zeal and devotion of the Grand-Duchess and Princess Wilhelm. — Sanitary movement in Bavaria.

In other parts of Germany engaged in the struggle, the efforts for succoring wounded soldiers were not less vigorous than in Prussia; only, the field of action being more restricted, and Prussian intervention having taken place from the beginning, these efforts could not manifest themselves in a manner as forcible and characteristic.

In Saxony, from the first news of the engagements that had taken place in Bohemia, several relief societies were voluntarily organized at Dresden, Leipzig, Chemnitz and Zittau. The women especially distinguished themselves by their eagerness in preparing lint, and placing at the disposal of the different committees which they had instituted, linen, refreshments and provisions.

When the trains of wounded arrived at Dresden, such a number of women presented themselves at the hospitals, that the medical officers had to intervene and refuse them access; they brought their offerings pell mell, moved by a noble sentiment of compassion, but without order and without discernment. And then, they demanded at times that the refreshments which they came in person, to offer to the wounded, should be given in preference either to the Saxons or the Austrians. Little by little order was establis-

hed, the service of voluntary relief centrali-
sed, and through the judicious efforts of the
President of the Saxon society, the excellent
and indefatigable General de Reitzenstein,
they were enabled to distribute advanta-
giously to all the wounded, the relief in
money and in kind which arrived abundantly
from all the districts of Saxony. The regular
hospital of Dresden having become insufficient, the military school and several other
establishments, particularly a large public
school, were converted into hospitals. Thus
transformed, the latter building seemed to me
to satisfy all exigencies, as a well aired and
well ventilated hospital.

The civil physicians of Dresden rivaled in
zeal the military ones of Prussia, and I doubt
whether wounded soldiers ever received
more intelligent and kinder attentions than
those in the hospitals of Dresden. As much

could be said of those in the hospital of
Zittau, where the ablest physicians of the
district came by turns to give their assistance
to the military surgeons.

If we now direct our attention to Southern Germany we there see also energetic endeavors to organize and centralize
the sanitary service upon the principles of
the Geneva convention, and even a certain
tendency to profit from the example given
by the United States Sanitary commission.
This tendency was manifested particularly
in Wurtemberg, where several local relief
societies were organized in the different
towns of the Kingdom, as soon as the conflict appeared inevitable. The service of
all these societies was centralized at Stuttgart under the direction of the *Sanitaets-
Verein*, an international society that was
placed under the direct patronage of the

Queen. There was, besides, a great enthusiasm in all classes of the population,
on account of the energetic impulsion gi- ✕
ven to the movement by both the King
and Queen; indeed it could hardly be
otherwise, since Wurtemberg had been one
of the first powers to sign the Geneva
Convention.

The Queen manifested in this underta- ✕
king a continued and commendable acti- ✕
vity. It was she, who so to speak, ini-
tiated the country in this humane work.
By her efforts, meetings were inaugurated at Stuttgart and in the principal
towns of the country, in which all classes
of society were made acquainted with the
aim and utility of relief societies. And
when the conflict had commenced and
hospitals were established for receiving the
wounded, the Queen did not fail in the

duty which she had voluntarily imposed
upon herself, but went frequently to stimulate by her presence the courage of the
patients, as well as the zeal of those who
had spontaneously offered themselves to
nurse them.

Seldom have we heard expressed, upon
the part that sanitary institutions are destined to perform in time of peace and
war, more elevated and just views than
those which the Queen was pleased to
communicate to us, when we had the
honor of conversing with her about the
results accomplished by the United States
Sanitary Commission. Never, said she one
day to us, had she experienced a sentiment of greater satisfaction than when,
having recognized how many services woman could render to humanity by taking
part in the Sanitary movement, she had

consecrated herself to the mission of actively propagating the sanitary reform in
her Kingdom.

Through the concurrence of all those
who, by their position or knowledge, could
influence the population, the resources of
the Sanitary Society rapidly augmented,
and during the short campaign in which
the troops of Wurtemberg were engaged, it
was enabled to render important services
by sending relief of every kind, as well as
male and female nurses, to the field hospitals established at Tauberbischofsheim and
the neighboring villages, after the bloody
battles which had taken place upon the banks
of the Mein. It even sent assistance to the
wounded of Bohemia, the hospitals of Vienna,
of Berlin, and of Munich. In the Grand-
Duchy we noticed an activity not less intelligent, and an excellent organization of the

international Society of Relief. But what
is curious and especially to be observed, is that in the Grand-Duchy it was,
as in the United States, women who first
had the generous thought of founding a
society of relief to the wounded.

As early as 1859, the *Badischer Frauenverein*, an association of ladies of the country of Baden, was organized at Carlsruhe,
through the initiative of the Grand-Duchess
Louise, with the object of succoring the
wounded during a war which seemed im-
minent at that period. Although the threa-
tened scourge was diverted, the association,
which had spread throughout the country,
continued its activity by adapting itself to
the less imperious exigences of peace,
without however abandoning its original
purpose. The central committee sitting
at Carlsruhe under the Presidency of the

Grand-Duchess, and having under its direction seventy-four collateral committees in the country, instituted, in 1861, a work which we could not sufficiently recommend to the attention of other Sanitary Societies; it founded Schools for the nurses to be employed in taking care of sick and wounded soldiers.

These female nurses are instructed in the hospitals of Carlsruhe, Pforzheim, and Mannheim. I see in an interesting work which Her Royal Highness has forwarded me, that these devoted women, after an apprenticeship of three months under the vigilant eye of physicians who give them daily theoretical and practical teaching, undergo an examination, and the central committee gives them certificates according to their capacities. When they have terminated their instruction, those who return

home in the city or country remain nevertheless under the direction of the local
Sanitary committee. A part of the nurses
stay in the hospitals where they perfect
themselves. Lastly some are employed in
an establishment at Carlsruhe, founded
by the Society, and nurse the sick at home
gratuitously in time of peace.

Such was the situation of this relief
Society when the international Convention
of Geneva took place, and to which the
Grand-Duchy of Baden was one of the first
adherents. The end proposed to be accomplished had already been foreseen
by the Society of the ladies of Baden;
it had even already organized one of the
branches of service most strongly recommen-
ded to the congress of Geneva. So that there
was no necessity of creating in the Grand
Duchy a new association especially char-

ged to represent the international convention.

But, when in the month of July 1866,
the hope of preserving peace had disap-
peared, the Grand Duchess Louise proposed
to the minister of war to intrust to the
Society, over which she presided, the functions of an International Society; this demand having been accorded without hesi-
tation by the Grand-Ducal Government,
the *Badischer Frauenverein* became from
that time one of the International Societies of Relief to the wounded, and it
must be admitted that, during the war,
it constantly proved how well its mission
was understood and has most worthily
fulfilled the noble duties intrusted to it.

From the time when the Baden troops
first began to experience the fatigues of for-
ced marchs, even before they had engaged

in the combats of the Mein and Tauler,
the international society under the Presidency of the Grand Duchess ably seconded
by the Princess Wilhelm displayed a continued activity.

To stimulate the interest of all, the
Grand Duchess accompanied by the Princess was seen to labor with the other
ladies of the committee; both overlooking
with extreme attention and solicitude the
operations of the society. On this account
relief in abundance reached the army from
the commencement of the campaign; first
cigars, eatables, and refreshments of all
kinds were sent; but after the engagements
of the 25th and 28th July, in which the Baden division had taken part, the central
committee of Carlsruhe forwarded to Wertheim and Tauberbischofsheim a number
of its female nurses, who rendered eminent

services in the ambulances or temporary
hospitals where wounded Prussians, Ba-
varians, Wurtembergians and Badoises were
lying side by side. " They fulfilled " says
the work I have cited " their arduous duties
to the full satisfaction of the physicians and
the wounded, and succeeded in conquering
the distrust which they encountered on their
arrival. Some of them belonged to the hig-
Kest classes of society. Besides, the material services which they rendered, their
excellent influence full of gentleness, the
order which they knew how to organize
in the small hospitals committed to their
care, and the consolation which they dif-
fused in the hearts of the suffering, show
of what great importance it is that women, whose education places them above
the ordinary level, should consecrate themselves to the care of the hospitals. The

assistant surgeons who had to do the heavy work of attending the wounded, too difficult for woman's hand, gained much by association with the lady nurses and fulfilled their difficult duties with greater care and consideration ".

The resources which the association possessed, by reason of the emulation that the central committee, had inspired in the country, were so considerable that at the end of the campaign it had still vast supplies in its possession, although it had forwarded considerable assistance to be distributed in the military hospitals of Bohemia, Vienna and Bavaria.

In Bavaria also the sanitary movement was considerable, and there too were associations of women especially who organized the service of relief to the wounded ; and, by the active intervention of these associations, the physicians of the Bavarian army, after the affair of Kissingen, had at their disposal a large quantity of lint, linen, bandages and instruments, at the same time that refreshments and provisions of every kind were sent to the hospitals.

After having exhibited the efforts which were tried in Prussia and southern Germany for nursing and succoring the wounded, I think I can truly say that nearly everything was done it was possible to do in a campaign which scarcely lasted three months, and I will add that, in an international point of view, all the obligations contracted by the signers of the Genevese convention were scrupulously fulfilled, particularly in Prussia and the grand-duchy of Baden.

CHAPTER IX

The *Patriotischer Damenverein*. — Princess de Schwarzenberg places her palace at the disposition of the ladies association. — Devotion of Madame de Lowenthal. — The *Patriotic Society* renders
great services to the army. — The *Holzhospital*. — Heroic conduct of two women.

Now what has been done in Austria? Here
we find ourselves as it were upon quite
different ground ; for it is no longer a question of national duties, and of the neutraliza-
tion of hospitals. Indeed it will be remembered that, for special reasons the Austrian
government had refused to sign the treaty of
Geneva. But what would it have done if
the fortune of arms had been favorable to

it; if, instead of leaving innumerable sick
and wounded in the hands of Prussia, it had
been called upon to provide for at the same
time, both its own wounded and a number
equally as considerable of Prussians? Would
it have been in condition to fulfil in a complete and irreproachable manner a task so
heavy? It must not be forgotten that Prussia
was enabled to fulfil everywhere and to the
end, towards numberless sick and wounded,
the difficult task imposed by victory itself,
not only by means of the superior organization of its military medical service, but especially through the spontaneous and continued
cooperation of sanitary associations; and I
will add that the force and grandeur of such
institutions consisted in their having an international character which enlisted their
sympathies alike for friends and enemies.

After these preliminary reflections, which

I cannot refrain from, having been upon
the theatre of events when the two armies
were still under arms, I will state that at
the close of the disasterous campaign, energetic and persevering efforts were made at
Vienna and in a large portion of the empire
to provide for the sick, and supply by the
free effort of individuals, what in the sanitary service of the army had seemed in-
complete and defective.

After the battle of Sadowa, most of the
wounded who had not been abandoned to
the care of the Prussian army were transported to Prague and Vienna; the first having
been left in the hands of Prussian physicians,
public solicitude was directed principally to
the multitudes of wounded in the capital.

From the beginning of hostilities an association which had already been in operation
during the campaign of Holstein, reentered

into active service with increased vigor and under a new form.

It was called the *Patriotischer Damen-verein*, patriotic society of ladies; as soon as war was determined upon, it placed itself under the presidency of princess Scharzen-berg, and appealed to all persons in the em- \
pire known for interesting themselves spe-cially in works of public benevolence, in order to engage them to participate in the association and accord it their earnest coö-peration. The first reunion of the associated ladies took place at the princess' residence and numbered only twenty seven persons, a few days later however a second meeting assembled forty, who obligated themselves to procure a thousand florins each for the society. These ladies exerted themselves with so much zeal and devotion that, shortly af- ✗
ter this second reunion, the society had at

its command a sum of one hundred and ten
thousand florins instead of the forty-eight
thousand which it had asked for. When the
trains of wounded arrived, the emperor placed
at the disposition of the *Patriotischer Damen-
verein*, two physicians, 'one of his palaces in
Hungary to be used as a hospital, and surgical instruments; while the sisters of charity,
ever present where there are sick to be cared
for, offered their services to the association.

Thus it was that the association of Austrian
ladies became one of the principal sanitary
societies of Austria, and rendered great services to the country, under the presidency of
a distinguished woman who had given up
to the society for hospital purposes, her
handsome palace, with its riding house and
stables. This lady undertook besides, the
lighting and warming of the establishment,
so that the association was charged only

with the expense of feeding the sick and
wounded. It could consequently dispose of
its funds more freely in favor of the sick
and convalescent. The society gave to each
convalescent, leaving the hospital Schwarzenberg which contained one hundred and
twenty beds, ten florins, and to those who
had suffered amputation of limbs, it gave
from one hundred and fifty to two hundred
florins; while to the officers, who left the
château before being entirely reestablished,
it delivered, according to circumstances,
four hundred and fifty and even six hundred
and fifty florins. Notwithstanding these libe-
ralities it still possessed sufficient capital to
assure to soldiers who had undergone grie-
vous operations, a life income of sixty florins.

But the solicitude of the ladies of this association was not confined alone to the
Schwarzenberg-hospital; even before the

last sick of this temporary establishment were transferred to the hospital of the order of Saint François, one of the members, the Baroness de Lowenthal, whose indefatigable exertion was the admiration of the population, had already called the attention of the society to this institution sustained by the liberality of the Imperial family; and which the emperor Maximilian had endowed with a sum of twenty one thousand florins. In this hospital, of the order of Saint François, Madam de Lowenthal by the attentions which she gave to the wounded, and especially by the manner in which she lavished them, stimulated a laudable emulation among the hospital employees, and again proved the happy influence always exercised in such circumstances by the presence of ladies belonging to the higher classes of society. If this society of ladies rendered good services, by reason of the devotion of its members, the *Patriotic Society*, from which women were excluded, was the one, of all the Austrian institutions organized and in operation during the war, which most resembled, in its organization and manner of operating, the American society. It had its central committee at Vienna, and local associations in most of the cities of the empire. It selected its members among men of readiness and willingness in all classes of society; and, like the sanitary associations of Prussia and the United States, it had organized volunteer hospital corps, who were in waiting at the principal railway stations to give the first attentions to the wounded who arrived, and distribute refreshments among them. Under the firm and able direction of its president, Prince Colloredo-Mansfield, this association, sprung from the free concurrence of the po-

pulation, rendered such important services
to the army, that, one of the first measures
of archduke Albert when he had taken command of the army of the North, was to make
sure of its cooperation.

When, some time after the battle of Sa- ✗
dowa, I visited the Austrian sanitary establishments, the hospitals of Vienna were
crowded with wounded, and most of them,
being insufficiently aired and lighted, encouraged a very great mortality.

One hospital however contrasted advanta-
geously with the others, by its cleanliness,
the disposition of its halls, and its good ventilation. Yet it was an improvised hospital,
called at Vienna the *Holzhospital*, because it
had been established in a wooden edifice,
destined for the agricultural exhibition which
took place at the Prater. This hospital was
intrusted to a ladies society under the presi-

dency of Madam Ida von Schmerling. Founded
the 20 *th* of June, this society, called *Damen
Comite*, had about fifty members. Some of
these established themselves in the hospital
confided to their care. They had a difficult
task to discharge, for there were in the
large hall alone of the building more than
five hundred sick to provide for. This establishment with a single story well aired and
lighted, reminded me forcibly of the wooden
hospitals such as were constructed in the
United States.

The immense influence exercised upon the
means of treatment by a proper ventilation
in the hospitals, is demonstrated by the fact
that in the establishment of the Prater, there
were but twelve cases of cholera, only two
of which proved fatal, while the epidemic
raged cruelly in the other hospitals. But a
fact still more striking is, that, out of five

thousand wounded treated in that establishment, only sixty-two were lost. Besides, only
two cases of mortification were observed and
cases of *pyæmia* were very rare. It is proper
here to add that the director of this hospital,
Doctor Abl, constantly gave proof of a zeal
and intelligence beyond all eulogy.

The members of the *Damen-Comite*, serving in this establishment, rivaled each other
in devotion ; yet when the epidemic broke out
there, their courage gave way. One after another they withdrew from the hospital until at
last there remained only two undaunted women whom nothing could cause to abandon
the post of honor which they had freely and
spontaneously accepted. I think it advisable here to mention the names of these
noble women. They were Madame Anna Stolz
and Mademoiselle Pelz. Left alone after the
retreat of their associates, these brave la-

dies exhibited courage and devotion in every
trial, occupied as they were for several weeks
in nursing the suffering, or cooking for two
or three hundred persons.

We see that acts of devotion in the cause
of humanity were not wanting in Austria ;
here, as in the rest of Germany, the populations contributed their offerings in order to
succor those who had been wounded in battle. The Austrians resident in France, thanks
to the active intervention of Madam the Prin- ✝
cess of Metternich, sent forward considerable
shipments to the relief societies of Vienna ;
while more than one hundred and thirty
packages were shipped in like manner from
Brussels to the same destination. Still, I repeat, the Austrian Sanitary institutions were
wanting in that cooperative character which
was the glory of similar enterprises organized in the United States and in Germany.

CHAPTER X

THE ITALIAN SOCIETY OF RELIEF TO THE WOUNDED

Medical society of Milan, under the impulsion of its president, organizes the first local Relief Society. — Appeal of this association
to Italy. — Committee of the Milanese Society recognized as central committee of the Italian Society of Relief to the wounded.
At the time of war the Florentine committee establishes itself as
central committee of the societies situated South of the Pô. —
Discussions following this incident. — Services rendered by the
Italian Society of Relief to the wounded.

If, in Austria, in spite of the incontestable
energy and enthusiasm of a portion of the
population, the Relief societies, from the fact
of their not being based upon a principle of
reciprocity, were lacking in that vigor and
initiative which the societies of Prussia,
Saxony, and Southern Germany manifested,
we meet again in Italy, although under a

different form, this same enthusiasm, this same power of popular initiative, thanks to the foresight and activity of the Italian Society of Relief to the wounded.

At the conference of Geneva, the Italian members took an active part in the debates, and the King of Italy was one of the first to adopt the agreement emanàting from those deliberations. As soon as the project of the convention had been determined, the medical society of Milan, under the inspiration of its president, Doctor Castiglioni, named a commission charged with preparing the statutes of a Relief society. This commission engaged with spirit, in the accomplishment of the task committed to it, and, on the 15 *th* of June 1864, the Milanese committee of the Italian Association of Relief for sick and wounded soldiers was constituted. This was not only the first Italian committee

of the kind, but, in general, one of the
first societies organized upon the principles of the Genevese convention. To jus-
tify its name of Milanese committee of the
Italian Society, a name which indicated
that it was only a member of a Society
more vast and important, the committee
of Milan made a spirited appeal to all the
medical societies of Italy, urging them to
follow its example and build up relief societies. At the same time that it communicated its statutes to the Medical Societies, it
published them, and invited citizens of all
classes to give their cooperation in the projected work. This appeal was heard; relief
societies were organised at Bergamo, Como,
Cremona, Pavia, and Monza; these local associations adopted the statutes of the Milanese
committee, and with unanimous consent
recognized as central committee of the Italian

Society of relief for the wounded, that of Milan
tan, which had had the good fortune of inaugurating the international sanitary movement
in Italy.

The entire work was placed under the patronage of King Victor-Emmanuel, and actually under the presidency of Doctor Castiglioni, the efficient president of the Milanese
committee, of which the Prince Royal was
honorary president. From the outset, the Society busied itself actively in its organization
and with the means of procuring resources in
kind and in money, in order to be ready to
fulfil its task should troublous times arrive.

The central committee, by reason of its
foresight and prudence found itself ready to
accomplish worthily the duties incumbent
upon it, when the events of **1866** happened
to bring into play all the energies of Italy. At
the approach of the danger several other

relief associations were founded in localities
where their organization had been neglected
during peace; and all these societies, those of
Ancona, Leghorn, Naples, Ferrara, Plaisance,
Turin, and Florence, operated in conjunction
with the Milanese committee, which they
considered as the central committee of the
association. Still at the very period when the
war broke out, an incident occurred which
sensibly touched the friends of a work that
was going, before the eyes of the whole nation, to test its power and decide a question
strongly controverted then in Italy : namely,
that of knowing if relief organized by the free
concurrence of the citizens could really produce the grand results expected of it. The
incident to which I make allusion, was the
proposition to give to the society two centers
of operation, one of which would remain at
Milan, and the other reside in the committee

of Florence. The partisans of this duality supported it by considerations which were not
wanting in strength and actuality. They al-
ledged that if the enemy crossed the Pô, the
communications of the Milanese committee
with southern Italy would be compromised;
but that so long as this event was not realized,
it was useful to have a center of action at Milan situated nearer the theatre of operations.

On the other hand the opponents of this
proposition, observed how dangerous it was
to introduce a schism in the administration of the society, at the very moment
when it should exhibit the extent of its
power; and to better demonstrate the pro-
priety of having only one central committee,
whatever might be the number of local
societies, or the importance of the work,
they remembered that the Sanitary Commission of the United States, which had

counted thirty thousand committees, and
had possessed riches to the amount of one
hundred and twenty-five millions of francs,
had, notwithstanding, never more than one
central committee : that established at Washington. These considerations should necessarily present themselves forcibly to
every mind; but there was still an objection not less weighty to oppose to the
measure proposed, and that was, as remarked by Doctor Castiglioni, since the
Milanese committee had already been recognized by all the other local societies
as the only central committee, it would
evidently then generate confusion in the
society at the very moment of action, to introduce this duality.

After lengthy discussions, and in spite of
the opposition of several societies, it was
finally arranged in such a manner that the

committee of Milan remained the center and the representative of the Italian Society, in relation with the International committee of Geneva. But in Italy it operated in reality, during the war, only as central committee of the local societies situated beyond the Pô; while by the very force of circumstances those of central and southern Italy assembled around the Florentine committee. Yet, although forming two centers, the two committees of Milan and Florence remained united in close relations, and their actions were always concerted in such a manner, that the relief service did not suffer by their common independence.

During the whole war the Italian Relief Society exhibited a remarkable activity and intelligence. In all the provinces of the Kingdom, but particularly in those of the center and North, there was an enthusiasm

and an emulation which did not cease
for a single day. The physicians, distinguished themselves by their zeal and readiness to enlist under the glorious banner
of the Society. During the days of Cus-
tozza, they were seen upon the field of
battle succoring the wounded, and, faithful to the mission of the Society, attending
Italians and Austrians indiscriminately.
The ambulance service of the Society also
was very well organized. The employees
of each division of the service, consisted
of a superior Sanitary officer, two assistant
sanitary officers, an administrator chosen by
preference from the clergy, a chief nurse
and eight assistants. The material consisted
of the flag of the International Society, ambulance satchels, medicine chests, litters so
arranged as to be used as tents when required, plain litters, sacks, bottles, and

10

goblets in wood, to be used by the wounded for drinking, cases of surgical instruments, and several varieties of baskets, for
carrying these objects in carriages or on
horseback. The ambulances of the Society
rendered a great service to the regular army
and to the volunteer corps; and the assistance in provisions and linen, which
the committees of Florence and Milan distributed in the hospitals, prove in a striking manner that all classes of Italian
society had also understood the grand role
reserved for individual initiative, when it
became a question of succoring the wounded
and cheering the victims of war. And
here, as elsewhere, it was the women especially, who by their courage, their energy,
and devotion, aided the Relief Society to
do all that it accomplished At Milan, Florence, Turin, and Ferrara, they did not

confine themselves to delivering lint, bandages, compresses, and linen, but they were seen also, especially at Florence and Milan, constantly occupied in aiding the committees in the depots of those cities.

CHAPTER XI

CONCLUSION

Relief Societies in operation during the last war have not offered any marked progress or improvment upon the methods employed by the United States sanitary commission. — Utility of sanitary collections. — The author's American sanitary collection. — Russia's adhesion to the Geneva convention. — International exhibition of Societies of Relief for the wounded. — Happy results of this exhibition.

I have exposed as minutely as possible the organization of the international relief societies, which were in operation during the recent events in Germany and Italy, conspicuously mentioning, at the same time, the services they have rendered. I have expressed unhesitatingly on more than one occasion, the unfeigned admiration I had felt at the sight of the devotion of volunteer physicians and nurses, the good will of sovereigns, and the intelligence and activity of the committees placed at the head of these associations. But, if I were now asked what improvements, I have been able to observe in Germany and Italy, upon the work instituted as early as 1861 in America by the United States Sanitary Commission, I am compelled to acknowledge that I have no where seen a striking amelioration, an improvement worthy of being signalled, either in the organization of the material of the Ambulances, or in the personal composition of the Sanitary Societies. I will even say, and I certainly speak without prejudice or partiality, that it is regrettable that the experience acquired in the United States during four years of a murderous war, was not turned to better profit;

it is particularly lamentable that many of
the excellent measures employed by the
American Sanitary Commission were not
adopted by the relief Societies in Germany,
and lastly, that a good number of American
inventions appropriate to the service of Ambulances were not employed by the different
committees.

A long study of the sanitary question,
such as it appeared in America, having fa-
miliarized me with most of these inventions, I knew what services they had rendered the United States Commission, and
how much they had aided it, in the
accomplishment of its glorious, but laborious task. So that, as soon as the idea of
organizing analogous associations in Europe
had sprung up, and consequently long before the Austro-Prussian war, I decided
to assemble in a collection as complete as

possible, the numerous Sanitary apparatus
and objects whose utility had been acknowledged during the civil war, by the American Commission in circumstances as serious
if not more difficult than those produced by
the late European conflict. Having commenced, immediately after the close of the war in
the United States, to gather the elements of
this Sanitary collection, I was already in possession of a large number of useful and interesting appliances when war broke out in
Germany; so that at the time I went upon the
theatre of events, I made it my duty to call
the attention of competent men to such of
these inventions as, in my opinion, could be
immediately introduced in the Sanitary service of the relief Societies. These communications, I must confess, were everywhere favorably received, and I believe that if the war
had continued much longer, the associations

of the belligerent countries would have been necessarily brought to make an application of a large number of these apparatus.

The war terminated, I could not choose a more favorable moment for inaugurating the American Sanitary Collection of which I have spoken, than at the opening of the Universal Exhibition. It found there its natural place in the International Exhibition of the Societies of relief to the wounded, since the collection was destined to offer to the consideration of the public, the numerous and varied means by which the first and most extensive of relief Societies had been able to realize the great object it had in view.

The limit traced by me in commencing this work has already been reached, I should however feel that my duty was still undone, if before closing I did not observe

that, since the last war which so agitated
Europe, earnest and able efforts have been
made to popularize, in every country the
idea of international Societies of relief for
the wounded. The benefits which these
associations have spread broadcast during
war had at once, a first and grand result,
in opening the eyes of a Great Power
which up to that time had refused to sign
the convention of Geneva : I speak of
Austria.

To decide on the question, she had only to
compare what had been done in Prussia
with what her own sanitary service had realized, notwithstanding the patriotism and
good will of the population.

As to Russia, it could not escape the pene-
tration of the emperor Alexander, that, after
a proof so decisive, most of the objections
which had been raised against the expe-

diency and efficacy of sanitary societies were dissipated. So we may consider the adhesion of Russia as decided in principal, and the conversations I have had upon this subject at Saint Petersbourg with the highest authorities of the country leave no doubt as to the early and definitive adhesion of this power to the international treaty (1). Nor has the progress of the sanitary movement been limited to the old world. My *History of the United States Sanitary Commission* soon after its publication, was translated into spanish both in Brazil and Paraguay and extensively circulated, and I learn that during the unhappy war which still ravages those distant countries upon the banks of the Plata, Sanitary Commissions have been established and relief societies organised.

(1) While this work was in press, a personal communication from Prince Gortschatkoff tells me that Russia has officially adhered to the convention of Geneva.

Indeed this treaty having been adopted by Austria and by Russia, it may be said that the international sanitary work becomes one of the most popular philanthropic institutions not only of Europe, but of the world, and I believe that in order to fortify it, and furnish it with the means of accomplishing in a complete manner its noble mission, no more simple and ingenious measure could have been taken than to invite to an international exhibition all the Societies of Relief for the wounded, organized upon the basis of the Genevese convention.

Through the initiative of the central committee of the French Society, which made a stirring appeal to the societies of other countries, this idea, happy in every point of view, has been realized, and we must congratulate those devoted men on the zeal which they have manifested in organising the exhibition intrusted to their care.

I repeat it, this reunion of all which, in different countries, has been imagined for succoring the wounded soldiers, will have been the most fruitful among the numerous measures adopted up to this time for propagating the international work of relief. Indeed from the comparative study of the objects, apparatus, and hospitals which have been employed in different countries, the best types may be chosen among the different models presented ; and useful inventions for sick or wounded soldiers will thus be adopted in countries where, perhaps, without this exposition, they would have long remained unknown.

But this international exhibition will have had still a result which, though less immediate, will not be less fortunate for the progress of the work whose success constitutes

the object of our most ardent wishes. I
allude to the good which must necessarily result for the work from the simultaneous presence at this exhibition of most of the eminent men who take an active part in the labors and operations of relief Societies both
in America and in Europe. These men by
exchanging their ideas, hopes and studies
will have mutually enlightened each other
upon the objects of their common solicitude,
and no doubt, returned to their firesides, will
have carried to their respective Societies new
and fertile ideas. As additional proof of
the reasonableness of this hope, we see
that from the intercourse of these men an
excellent idea has already been developed,
and one to which those who wish sincerely
the development of the sanitary work will
not refuse their concurrence. I allude to
the international conferences of the So-

cieties of relief for the wounded which took place during the Universal Exhibition.

In those international conferences of the relief societies of Europe and the United States, scientific questions were discussed from a sanitary point of view, and long sittings were consecrated to the study of serious improvements relating to the work. About 50 delegates, representing societies organised in different countries, took part in the interesting deliberations which characterised those international reunions, and obtained the following principal results :

A project for certain modifications in the text of the Geneva treaty of 1864 was unanimously adopted. This project, the exact text of which we give further on, could not fail to be favorably and unanimously accepted, since its principal aim was to make participators in the benefits of neutrality, those relief societies which were not in existence when the convention in vigor had established the principle of the neutrality of hospitals and their attendants.

Doubtless all the powers signing that treaty will readily and cheerfully give their assent to the modifications proposed by the late international assembly.

In order that the neutrality accorded, may be better appreciated and the result of the conferences fully understood I give below the complete text of the convention agreed upon.

TREATY

For the amelioration of the condition of wounded soldiers in the armies of the land and sea.

ARTICLE FIRST.

Ambulances, hospitals and all material, destined to aid the sick and wounded, upon land and sea, will be recognised as neutral, and as such, protected and respected by belligerents.

Under the enemy's authority they will still preserve their wages, etc.

This sanitary assistance will not be detained beyond the time required for the attention of the wounded, but the commander in chief of the victorious army or naval forces will decide when it may withdraw.

The sanitary and administrative service, as well as the wagons, ships and all material for the use of the wounded, will continue to operate upon the field of battle or in the waters where the combat has taken place, even after those places shall have been occupied by the victorious army or naval forces. However, the wounded removed shall remain in the hands of the conqueror. If the sanitary and administrative service should fail in the duties imposed by its neutrality, it shall be submitted to the laws of war.

ART. 4.

The members of the societies of Relief for wounded soldiers in the land and naval armies of every country, as also their auxiliary attendants and their material, are declared neutral.

The Relief societies will put themselves in direct communication with the head quarters of the armies or with the commandants of the naval forces, by means of representatives.

11

The Relief societies, in accord with their representatives at the head quarters of the land or naval forces, may send delegates who shall follow the armies or the fleets upon the theatre of war, and second the sanitary and administrative services in their operations.

Art. 5.

The inhabitants of the country, as well as volunteer hospital attendants or nurses, who shall aid the wounded, will be respected and protected.

The commandants in chief of the belligerent powers will invite, by a proclamation, the inhabitants of the country to succor the enemy's wounded, as if they belonged to a friendly army or marine.

Every wounded soldier received and cared for in a habitation will serve as a protection for it.

Every vessel charged with receiving the wounded or ship-wrecked will be protected under the colors mentioned in the following article n° 7.

Art. 6.

The sick or wounded soldiers will be received and nursed, regardless of their nationality. Every wounded person fallen into the hands of the enemy is declared neutral, and must be turned over to the civil or military authorities of his country, to be sent home when circumstances permit and the consent of the two parties is obtained.

The convoys of the health service, with the persons who direct them, will be protected by an absolute neutrality.

Art. 7.

A distinct and uniform flag and pavilion are adopted for the hospitals, ambulances, depots of supplies, and the convoys of the health service, in the land and marine armies. They must be, in every circumstance, accompanied with the national flag or pavilion.

A badge is likewise admitted for the neutral service.

This badge will be delivered exclusively by the military authorities, who will create for that purpose certain regulations.

Every person illegally carrying the badge will be subjected to the laws of war.

The flag, ship's colors, and the badge shall bear a red cross upon a white back ground.

Art. 8.

It Is the duty of the victorious army to over look, as much as circumstances permit, the soldiers fallen upon the field of battle, to protect them from pillage and bad treatment, and to bury the dead in strict conformity with sanitary prescriptions.

The contracting powers will take care that in time of war, every soldier is provided with a uniform and obligatory sign or mark suitable to establish his identity.

This sign shall indicate his name, place of birth, as well as the army corps, regiment and company to which he belongs. In case of death, this document must be taken off before burial and sent to the civil or military authority of the deceased's place of birth.

The lists of dead, sick, wounded and prisoners, shall be communicated as complete as possible, im· mediately after the engagement, to the commander of the enemy's army by a diplomatic medium.

In so far as the contents of this article are applicable to the marine and executable by it, they will be observed by the victorious naval forces.

Art. 9.

The high contracting powers obligate themselves to introduce in their military regulations the modifications become necessary by reason of their adhesion to the convention.

They will order the explanation of them to the land and naval troops in time of peace, and will see that they are included in the order of the day in time of war. The commanders in chief of the belligerent armies or navies will see to the strict observance of the convention, and will regulate for this purpose the details of its execution. The inviolability of the neutrality set forth in this convention must be guaranteed by uniform declarations, published in the military codes of the different nations.

Another question equally important was discussed and resolved by the conference. It became necessary to determine upon what basis should be founded the international centre of Relief societies. It was decided, in principle, that a superior international committee formed of the delegates of different societies should sit at Geneva, and that a sub-committee (international) having its head quarters at Paris should operate under the authority of the superior committee.

To give to the work at once a progressive and regular movement, a special commis-

sion was appointed to examine the propo-
sitions of the international committee of
Geneva.

The committee is composed of the following gentlemen :

Count Serurier, delegate of the French Committee.
Movnier, delegate of the Swiss Committee.
H. de Luck, chevalier of the Order of St. John of Jerusalem, and
delegate from the grand-Master of that order.
Count F. de Breda, delegate of the French Committee.
Dʳ Seitz, delegate of the Munich Committee.
Major Staaff, delegate of the Swedish Committee.
Van de Velde, delegate of the Antwerp Committee.
Dʳ Thoʳ. W. Evans, delegate of the United-States Committee.
Dʳ Ancona, delegate of the Italian Committee.
Dʳ Hahn, delegate of the Sanitary Society of Stuttgard (Wir-
temburg).
Theodore Vernes, treasurer general, delegate of the French
Committee.
Count de Luxbourg, delegate of the General Society of Bavaria.
Charles Bowles, delegate of the United-States Committee.
Dʳ P. Castiglioni, delegate of the Italian Committee, secretary.
Dʳ Piotrowski, delegate of the French Committee.
Dʳ Gadvin, secretary general, delegate of the French Committee.
Dʳ Shanzenbach, delegate of the general Society of Bavaria.
Dʳ Barbieri, delegate of the Committee of Italy.
Soriano-Fuertes, delagate of the Committee of Spain.
Dʳ Texeira d'Aragao, delegate of the Committee of Portugal.

The international conference having decided that it would award prizes and medals, these honors were accordingly distributed to the promoters, protectors and cooperators of the international work. It is perhaps to be regretted that they have been offered to persons, eminent without doubt, but who (as regards some at least) may be embarrassed by such marks of distinction and may even be, from various considerations, compelled to refuse to accept them.

From the preceeding pages it will be observed that much has been accomplished. Much still remains to be done through earnest effort and wise counsel, and I most sincerely trust that as an effective means of realising our hopes, these international conferences may be continued regularly after the Exhibition, both in France and other countries. May they multiplying, call upon the entire work the sympathy of every nation! Then, and then only the Relief Societies will succeed in fulfilling completely their mission : that of mitigating the horrors of war while awaiting the arrival of a more advanced civilization to extirpate the terrible scourge.

APPENDIX

AMBULANCE WAGONS

If the means of transport for the sick and wounded, have scarcely been improved in the presence of the many ameliorations introduced into the armies of Europe within the past few years, it must be attributed less to a feeling of indifference than to the almost insuperable difficulties which beset this subject.

The single fact that no Government has ever used an ambulance wagon which has not been a fair subject for the severest criticism, shows very clearly how many obstacles must be overcome before a positive excellence is reached.

An ordinary wagon, will certainly not furnish the most comfortable or the safest means of transportation for a severely wounded man, while a wagon admirably adapted to special cases, may be quite unsuitable for the more general services of a campaign.

The great question to decide is, how can the sick and wounded be best transported, most humanely and comfortably to themselves, as well as most conveniently and economically to the administration. For the system which shall·clearly contribute in the largest degree to the special interests of the individual, and at the same time to the more general interests of the army and the Government, must be accepted as the best attainable good, however imperfect it may seem.

Although it does not fall within my present purpose to enter into a detailed consideration of the different kinds of transport now employed in armies, a general examination of the previous question compels at least an allusion to some of the means best knownat present.

Stretchers, wheeled litters, *tablier*, etc., must be regarded as of secondary importance, their service being necessarily confined to the transportation of the wounded from where they may have fallen, to the ambulance wagons, or the temporary field hospitals, or to the movement, whenever it may seem desirable, of any sick or wounded man from one point to another in the immediate vicinity.

The *cacolets* and horse litters used by the French

army in Algeria, and in regions mountainous or in-
accessible to wheeled vehicles, must also be considered as limited in their employment strictly to the
circumstances which have created them and as indif-
ferent substitutes for superior means of transport.

The principal means of transport for the sick and
wounded must always be the ambulance wagon. Of
these wagons there are many different models now
in use in Europe — some with two and some with
four wheels — some intended to convey the wounded
only in a recumbent position, and others so constructed that the wounded may be carried either
recumbent or sitting. Nearly all these ambulance
wagons fail in several essential particulars. They are
without exception unnecessarily heavy and clumsy.
The French four wheeled ambulance weighs 950 ki-
lograms (1860 pounds) and the English and Italian
wagons weigh even more. The wheels of the English
ambulance are sufficiently solid for a gun carriage.
The Italian, French and Austrian ambulances have
wooden sides and ends, and are covered in some
instances with double wooden roofs ; in a word they
may be described as *omnibuses*.

In the construction of all these vehicles massi-
veness has apparently been regarded as something
indispensable. This is a serious mistake. Lightness
is so important a consideration that everything su-
perfluous to the comfort of the wounded, or not ab-

solutely necessary for their security, or the security
of the carriage itself, should be unhesitatingly rejected.

An ambulance should be so light as to be easily
and rapidly drawn by *two horses* anywhere it is
possible for a carriage to penetrate — across mea-
dows and fields as well as on macadamized roads.
In fact it should realise the idea expressed by the
word *volante*.

The difficulty of using the European ambulances,
except on well constructed public ways, is an objection fatal to them.

The ambulances used by the United States Government during the late American war, are, as regards
this great essential — lightness — the best which
have yet been constructed. The American four wheeled ambulances rarely exceeded 1250 lbs. in weight.
At the commencement of the war a large number
of ambulances (Triplers), weighing each about as
much as the four-wheeled French wagon, were furnished by the United States Government, but they were
abandoned after a few weeks trial. Four horses were
often insufficient to extricate them from the mud,
or pull them over roads rendered difficult by the
passage of wagon and artillery trains. Light four
wheeled carriages were soon adopted and it was
admitted universally, after four years experience,
that they were sufficiently strong for the special

service to which they were destined, and vastly su-
·perior to the heavy vehicles which they had suc-
cceded.

An ambulance should be so constructed as to turn
easily and safely within a circle whose diameter
should be but little greater than the length of the
wagon.

A most serious objection to the American ambulances is the difficulty and danger with which
they are turned. The objection is also applicable
to the English wagons. In the French, Italian and
Swiss ambulances the front wheels are low and pass
either partially or entirely beneath the body of the
carriage. This should always be the case, as the in-
crease of power unquestionably gained by high
wheels can by no means be an equivalent for the
serious inconvenience alluded to. Another point to
be considered is ventilation. The French, Austrian,
and Italian ambulances are in this respect particularly bad. The American plan of using for wagon
coverings enameled cloth or more commonly simple
cotton duck, is admirable not only in view of economy and lightness, but especially from the ease
with which the interior can be thrown open to the
light and air. The adequacy of these coverings to the
securing of the comfort of the patient in winter as
well as summer, their durability and impermeabi-
lity to rain have been abundantly proven in the

United States. Whether the unenameled cotton duck would prove equally durable in the more humid climates of Europe is a proper subject for experiment.

Ambulances should be so arranged as to carry men either recumbent or sitting. The French one horse ambulance can carry two men recumbent only. Even admitting the expediency of employing two or more forms of ambulance — lighter and heavier — in the same army, this principle of construction should be observed in each. The ease with which the principle can be adopted and the serious embarrassements which must frequently arise from a neglect of it are sufficient reasons for its acceptance.

The best form of ambulance must always be that with four wheels. This has been generally admitted, probably however rather in view of the larger capacity of the four wheeled vehicles than from a recognition of that jerky highly uncomfortable movement, resulting from any pace faster than a walk, which must always constitute a radical defect in the two wheeled ambulance. This fact particularly led to the total abandonment of this class of wagons by the United States Government soon after the commencement of the late war.

Having spoken of some of the more general rules to be observed in the construction of field ambulance wagons, it remains for me to consider the

internal arrangement best adapted to the transportation of sick and wounded men. In the first place
means should be taken to secure the severely sick
or wounded from shocks and concussions to the
largest degree practicable, by the employment of
stretcher mattresses furnished with springs similar
to those used in the English ambulances, or by fixed
springs upon which the mattresses may rest as in the
Howard ambulance. Again, the interior construction
should admit the ready loading and unloading of
the carriage. This is a most important subject and
one with reference to which there is the greatest
room for improvement even in the best models with
which I am acquainted. The severely wounded
should never, without a special reason be removed
from the litter (brancard) employed in carrying
them to the ambulance, but the interior of the
vehicle should be so arranged that the *brancard*
may be placed readily within it and be as readily
withdrawn whenever necessary. This end is very
well secured in the Howard Ambulance. It is to be
regretted however that Howard has not at the same
time remedied many of the inconveniencies resulting from the special arrangements he has adopted.
Not only should the loading and unloading be accomplished without unnecessarily disturbing the
wounded but it should be done easily by the attendants. In nearly all the wagons hitherto built, either

the body has been so high, or the door so narrow, or the steps so deficient or badly arranged, that it has been only with the greatest difficulty that a wounded man could be lifted up into the place he was to occupy.

These are necessarily general considerations.

The special interior arrangement must depend upon the size and proposed capacity of the wagon.

After a pretty extended investigation of this subject — an investigation which has to some extent been conducted on the field itself — I have come to the conclusion that an interior disposition as follows, if not the best possible, would at least be an improvement on any now employed.

Presuming as an indispensable preliminary that the wagon itself is sufficiently light to be easily drawn anywhere by two horses, I would have it so arranged that it might comfortably transport ten men sitting, besides the driver, or four men recumbent and two sitting.

The utility as well as the economy of being able to transport four men recumbent is almost too apparent to need discussion. Mr Sûs of New-York who first called the attention of the United States Government to this subject, and who is the real inventor of the ambulance now accepted as preferable to all others by the Medical Bureau, under the name of Rucker, has furnished us with

some most astonishing figures in which he shows
the enormous saving in wagons, horses, forage,
men, etc., which may be obtained by the general adoption of this system of transport. Sûs and
Rucker have both failed however, not only with
reference to points of exterior construction to which
we have before alluded, but also in the arrangement of their seats and mattresses to which there
are neither springs, handles or rollers[1]. The result
is, notwithstanding the excellence of the original
idea, that practically the difficulty of getting a
severely wounded man into a Rucker ambulance is
if possible exceeded by the difficulty of getting him
out. But how can these faults be remedied?

In the first place by dispensing altogether with the
upper mattresses which are clumsy and impracticable in the highest degree as mattresses, and when
folded as backs for seats, render these seats narrow and do not offer a single advantage which
might not be better gained by a light, simple and
permanent padding. In place of these upper mattresses I would use ordinary field stretchers
(French, English or American), the handles of

[1] It is true that in the model Rucker ambulance sent to the Exposition by the U. S. medical Bureau, there are handles to the lower
tier of mattresses. These mattresses are also supplied with india-
rubber wheels, which are however made so thin as to be easily bent
quite out of shape. In the model they are utterly worthless as regards
the purpose intended.

which should be received in strong india-rubber
loops, two to be attached to each side, two feet and
nine inches from the floor, two to a perpendicular
post in the middle of the wagon immediately behind
the seat of the driver, and two to a jointed iron
rod, which can be dropped when desired from the
center of the rear bow. This is substantially the
system of suspension employed with so much success by the Americans in their celebrated hospital
cars. The elasticity of the india-rubber will secure a
sufficient degree of comfort to the patient, while the
simplicity of the arrangement, and the possibility of
employing ordinary field stretchers as mattresses
constitute practical advantages of the highest importance.

In the second place, by adding to the seats of
the Rucker ambulance, which when opened are
to be used as mattresses upon the floor of the wagon, sliding handles, and small iron wheels which
when the mattresses are in position should rest upon
strong steel springs sunk in the floor of the vehicle
and flush with its surface.

I am aware that certain objections may be urged
against the employment of two tiers of couches in
an ambulance wagon, but it must be observed that
the arrangement for our upper tier is not fixed and
permanent but entirely supplementary, and inter-
feres in no way with the employment of the wagon

for the transport of two men should it at any time seem desirable to carry only two recumbent; but all who are acquainted with the frequently pressing necessities of the hospital service, must recognize the immense importance of any application which at a critical moment may double the capacity of the vehicle [1].

In order that the loading and unloading may be effected easily and rapidly by the attendants, the wagon from the floor to the roof should not be less than one and a half metres (4 feet 10 1/2 inches) high, should be furnished with a broad rear step, and two steps on each side in front, and the driver's seat should either be so low, or fold upon itself in such a way, as to furnish no obstacle to the attendant bearing the front end of the stretcher into the wagon, and asto permit him, after properly securing the handles of the stretcher to the rubber rings, to step to the ground from the front of the ambulance.

A place should be reserved for a water tank and a few indispensable stores, and there should be also a place either on the inside or outside of the wagon for two or more supplementary litters. But in the construction of an ambulance there is great danger

---

[1] In the accompanying catalogue page 200 will be found a more detailed description of an ambulance which has recently, been constructed upon the principles here presented.

of attempting to accomplish too much. A great many
ingenious expedients are constantly being suggested
for the increased comfort of the patient or the con-
venience of the attendant. There will always be dif-
ferences of opinion as to the relative value of such
improvements but many of them, even admitting
their importance, must be rejected or our system
will be found too complicated for the requirements
of field service.

The Italian ambulance of Locati, excellent in
many respects is an example of a too complicated
system.

In selecting an ambulance it seems to me, as
before observed, that the question should not be
what form of ambulance is that which will transport
individual soldiers or officers, sick or wounded,
with most comfort and least danger to themselves,
but what is that form or those forms which in view
of the various requirements of actual service will
fulfil best their specials functions and at the same
time best secure the general good of the whole
army.

Several of the wheeled litters proposed by Neuss,
Fischer, Gauvin and others, are unquestionably more
comfortable means of transport for a severely wounded man than any of the horse wagons now known,
and yet it would be in the highest degree unwise to
substitute to any considerable extent such litters for

wagons drawn by horses. The amount of transportation required for such litters and the number of men necessary for their special service, must forever preclude their general employment in the field. In this connection, I may allude also to the danger of forgetting the proper function of the stretcher mattresses which should accompany every ambulance. These should be considered essentially as mattresses and not as stretchers or litters The mattress should always be so constructed that it may be used as a stretcher if needed, but comparatively few stretchers should be furnished with the appliances necessary to an ambulance mattress, as during a campaign occasions for the use of the simple stretcher must continue to be vastly the most frequent, no matter to what extent we may adopt new systems of transport or improve our old ones.

Another important means of transport is that by rail, either by ordinary carriages or by carriages especially prepared, under the name of railway ambulances or hospital cars. The Americans, operating in a country traversed by more than 50,000 kilometres of navigable rivers, and more than 60,000 kilometres of railway, and impressed with the immense importance of reinvigorating, by a change of climate, their soldiers wasted or enfeebled by the diseases peculiar to hot and malarious districts, transported whole armies of men by steamboats and

railways to the convalescent camps and stations of
the North.

In this service the ordinary carriages were generally employed ; but the necessity of securing some
better means of transit for the severely sick and
wounded soon led them to the use of the so-called
hospital cars, which were simply the common American carriages with a special interior arrangement
permitting the suspension of litters in tiers on either
side of a central passage way, and furnished with
two or three cabinets for medicines, the preparation
of food, etc. In these carriages the severely wounded
were often transported several hundred miles without a change and with the greatest comfort to
themselves. One or two of these special cars were
generally found sufficient for a hospital train.

The European railway carriages are not as suscep-
tible of being readily converted into good hospital
cars as the American carriages, owing to their smaller
size and their division into several compartements.
Still it will be doubtless found not difficult to apply
to these cars every thing essential to the easy and
safe transit of the sick over long routes.

My remarks upon this most important subject
have necessarily been brief and fragmentary, still
if this expression of opinions, which have not been
hastily formed but are the results of a most careful
and laborious study, may in any way aid in the esta-

blishment of some more perfect system than is now in use my object will have heen attained.

From the committee of the International relief societies, which has been especially charged with the examination of all hospital material exhibited at the Exposition, we have much to hope, and I sincerely trust that, conducting its inquiries free from the prejudices of routine, and in that spirit of enlightened criticism which is the glory of our epoch, some progress may be made, some amelioration effected, in the practical conduct of one of the most important branches of military service.

———

Penetrated with the idea that the Sanitary Commission of the United States, by mitigating the horrors of war, had resolved one of the most urgent questions of modern time, I thought it just and proper to acquaint the European public with the great number of ingenious inventions made in America in view of ameliorating the condition of sick and wounded soldiers.

As early as the year 1865 I decided to assemble in a collection and at my own expense, the products of these inventions which had enabled the Sanitary Commission to obtain its wonderful results.

In order to realize this project, I addressed myself to my countrymen in America. After having explained to them the aim I was pursuing, I urged them to assist me in an enterprise, the humanitarian and patriotic tendency of which was evident. In addressing myself to all American inventors or manufacturers, my object was to decide every one to produce his invention, so that in my collection might be exhibited such articles as would have perhaps other wise remained unknown or unnoticed.

However my address had no appreciable result; and the enterprize which with the expected contribution or assistance, would have been rather an easy work, became now a difficult task. If I nevertheless succeeded in assembling a collection as complete as possible, I am indebted for it to the intelligent and most active cooperation of my friend Dr Edward A. Crane, who went out to the United-States, in order to select there such articles as were suitable to the object I had in view.

The Universal Exhibition afforded the best opportunity for the inauguration of this sanitary collection; its natural place being in the international exhibition of the Societies of Relief for wounded soldiers (*exposition internationale des sociétés de secours aux blessés*).

Since the day when it was placed in a distinct and special building in the Champ de Mars, there has been, I think, no military surgeon and even no sovereign who has visited the grand Exhibition without paying a visit to the collection and giving a tribute of sincere admiration to the deeds of the American Sanitary Commission.

When the work of the United States Sanitary

Commission was examined by the Imperial Commission, the collection exhibited in the Champ de Mars, was considered as belonging to the Xth group, and the large golden medal or *Prix d'honneur* was awarded to it, as one of the noblest of those institutions private or public, which have advanced human welfare or mitigated human suffering.

I was appointed to receive the medal, which was delivered to me by the Emperor in the solemn assembly of the 1^{rst} July, and now hold this medal at the disposal of the United States Commission[1].

Other prizes, medals, and mentions, have been likewise decreed to the American collection by the Imperial Commission and the international Societies of Relief. Here are the lists.

FROM THE IMPERIAL COMMISSION.

Silver medal.

G. TIEMANN et Co. — Surgical instruments.

Bronze medals.

Dr E. HARRIS. — Railway ambulance.
Dr HUDSON. — Artificial limbs.

Honorable mention.

Dr HOWARD. — Ambulance.

---

[1] Since the above was written I have delivered to the Reverend Dr Bellows, President of the U. S. Sanitary Commission, the medal alluded to.

Gold medals.

Rev Dr BELLOWS.
Dr THOMAS W. EVANS.

Silver medal.

The Relief Committees.
Dr E. A. CRANE.

Bronze Medal.

The Secretaries of the Committees.

TO EXHIBITORS.

Silver Medals.

BORDEN. — Preserved food.
TIEMANN. — Surgical instruments.
DUNTON. — Medicine basket.
PEROT. — Medicine wagon.

Bronze Medals.

Dr E. HARRIS. — Railway ambulance.
G. AUTENREITH. — Medicine wagon.
Ambulance wagon.
J. BRAINARD. — Ditto.
Instruments of Surgery.
Dr J. CROSBY. — Bed for sick persons.
Dr J. Q. COLTON. — Apparatus for protoxide of azote.
Dr GURDON-BUCK. — Fracture apparatus.
A. M. DAY. — Splints.
Dr HUDSON. — Orthopedy.
Dr LANGER. — Extension bed.
Dr LATTA. — Fracture bed.
Madame PETITEAU. — Bed for the wounded.
PINNER. — Ambulance kitchen.
M. W. RICHARDSON. — Hospital tent.
F. S. STEVENS. — Bed-table.
M. WALTON. — Officers tent.
F. P. WOODCOCK. — Horse litter.

Independently of these rewards an honorable mention has been specially accorded to us by the Minister of war, for services rendered to armies in campaign, and a prize (*hors concours*) of five hundred francs has been decreed to the author for an ambulance which he has constructed upon a new plan.

This sum has been turned over to the international Society.

Indeed so attractive a subject of interest has this collection proved to be as well as so efficient a means of disseminating useful and practical knowledge, that with the close of the Exhibition, I have been encouraged to enlarge it, and at the same time to give to it an international character by making it a permanent repository of what ever, in the hospital service of armies, shall have been invented or employed for the purpose of ameliorating human suffering.

Since this Essay on Sanitary Institutions during the austro-prussian-italian conflict was published in French, I have received many evidences of the importance which competent judges attribute both to the questions I have treated in this book and to the collection I have exhibited in the Champ de Mars. Among numerous letters addressed to me on that subject, I shall only communicate a few, which have seemed to me to possess, either from the distinguished position of the writer or from the value of the opinions expressed, something more than an interest personal with myself.

TO THOMAS W. EVANS M. D.

SURGEON TO THE EMPEROR OF THE FRENCH

Coblence, 20ᵗʰ July 1867.

« During my sojourn in Paris I received your most important work, — a memorial of the war of 1866. I thank you heartily for it. As a competent judge you have, by publishing this book, once more given a proof of the zeal and the charity which are your motives, and of which your Sanitary American collection is the purest manifestation. May a durable peace be the reward of your noble efforts to mitigate the horrors of war.

« AUGUSTA. »

Queen of Prussia.

Paris, Polytechnic School, 15ᵗʰ July 1867.

« Dear Doctor, EVANS,

« I received yesterday your new work : The Sanitary Institutions during the *austro-prussian-italian conflict*, which I read without once leaving it off. Your book, by making known the organization and function of the Prussian Society of relief, assures, in my opinion, the success of similar societies in France and in Europe in future wars.

« Notwithstanding the Convention of Geneva, we had in France no real faith in the efficiency of private societies concurring with the official action of the department of war. The example you quote proves sufficiently that private societies of relief to wounded soldiers, without being in any way an obstacle, are on the contrary indispensable auxiliaries to the official organization in circumstances in which this organization is insufficient.

« Without alluding to many other questions treated in your book, I will add that I consider it a work destined to do great service to humanity. I thank you for having afforded me the great satisfaction of reading it, and remain,

« Yours very truly,

« FAVÉ,

Aide de camp of the Emperor and Governor of the Polytechnic School.

Mainau, grand-duchy of Baden.

Dr THOMAS W. EVANS,

I regret very much not to have been able to send you sooner inclosed notes, though they have been written as soon as it was possible to know even approximatively the figures they contain.

I hope they will be useful for the noble work to which you have devoted your attention and your interest.

LOUISE.

Grand-Duchess of Baden.

Paris, 25ᵗʰ August 1867.

DOCTOR THOMAS W. EVANS.

Sir,

I have read with great interest your work upon assistance given to the sick and wounded during the recent wars in America, Germany and Italy. Men who consecrate themselves to the alleviation of the sufferings of humanity will find therein precious information, and I cannot too highly congratulate you on the noble devotion and great sagacity with which you have sought and promulgated that information.

Believe me, doctor,

Yours very respectfully,

Marshal CANROBERT.

Paris, 16ᵗʰ August 1867,

DOCTOR THOMAS W. EVANS.

Sir,

Several journals have spoken of the exhibition of the international Societies of Relief to wounded soldiers of the land and marine armies. They have well comprehended the object of the work, but have not generally sufficiently remarked the incontestable superiority of the means employed in the United States.

The ambulance wagon, vehicles, alimentary preserves, proofs of attentions of every kind, all bear the stamp of the most enlightened patriotism, and of the importance which the Americans attach to the preservation of human life and the alleviation of the inevitable evils of war.

You may be proud of the success, and I am happy to express to you my admiration for those inspirations of a charity which has encountered no limits, because it has been recognised in America that the asssistance to be given to the glorious victims of the battle field must be proportioned to the nature of the sacrifice.

The country has considered itself bound to pay a sacred debt, and has not assimilated this assistance

13

to that assured by charity to the poor received in civil hospitals.

Believe me, sir,

Yours very respectfully,

H. CHENU,
Principal Army Physician.

Austrian Embassy. — Paris, 26th February, 1867.

THOMAS W. EVANS,
DOCTOR IN MEDICINE

I take great pleasure in informing you that the Emperor my August Sovereign has received the works, relating to military Hygiene and the Sanitary Commission of the United States, which you have requested me to present to him.

Appreciating the philanthropic thought which has guided you in researches and studies of which these publications are the meritorious fruit, and recognizing the beneficial influence your labors are destined to have upon military Medicine and Hygiene, His Imperial Majesty has charged me to return to you his sincere thanks for these interesting volumes, to which a place has been assigned in his private library. Yours very respectfully,

Prince DE METTERNICH.

Munich (Bavaria), 4ᵗʰ February 1865

DOCTOR THOMAS W. EVANS.

Sir,

I had the honor to receive your interesting publication upon the United States Sanitary Commission.

The king and the queen mother, to whom transmitted two copies, have requested me to ex press to you their thanks. I embrace this occasion to send you my own thanks for the copy you had the kindness to design for me.

Accept, my dear sir, the expression of my highest consideration,

The counselor of State,

FR. VON PFISTERMEISTER.

The Hague, 15ᵗʰ January 1865.

DOCTOR THOMAS W. EVANS. — PARIS.

Dear Sir,

Her Majesty the Queen of Holland has received the copy of your work upon the United States Sanitary Commission, which you have been so good as to send her.

Very sensible of this attention, I am requested by Her Majesty to express to you her thanks, the more sincere, as through your labors she is enabled to appreciate the immense services rendered by that institution.

Her Majesty most earnestly desires the development of a work which soon, she is convinced will extend its benefits to every civilised nation.

Accept on this occasion, Sir, the assurances of my esteem and believe me.

Your very respectfully,

W. J. WECKHERLIN.

Counsellor of State.

Paris, 17ᵗʰ October 1867.

Doctor Thomas W. Evans,

The visit which I made this morning to your sanitary collection has deeply interested me. I wish you to know this, and also to thank you for your kindness in furnishing me with useful information concerning the principal objects which compose it.

I wish also to tell you, how sensible I am of the persevering efforts and sacrifices you are making in behalf of the great work of the International commission of succor for the wounded.

I remember what you wrote me at the time you

sent me your book upon the United States Sanitary Commission, as well as my own reply. I see with an agreeable satisfaction that our mutual aspirations were well founded — that what was then a hope has to-day become a reality for the welfare of humanity.

Believe me, my dear doctor, with the sincerest thanks.

Yours,

SOPHIE,

Queen of Holland.

Paris, 13th May 1862.

DR. THOMAS W. EVANS,

In reply to your letter — I thank you for the information which you have given me with reference to the organisation and useful labors of the United States Sanitary Commission.

That institution has awakened my liveliest interest, and I gladly believe that at no distant day, many associations, animated by the same spirit of charity and humanity, will be organised every where, to give succour to the wounded and the sick — to friends and enemies alike.

EUGÉNIE,

Empress of the French.

CATALOGUE OF ARTICLES

UNITED STATES

SANITARY COLLECTION

OF

Dr THOMAS W. EVANS

CLASS I. — AMBULANCES.

GROUP FIRST. — Ambulances of Transport.

Number
of Articles.

1.

N° 1.   An Ambulance; known as Howard's Ambulance ; made from plans furnished by Dr. B. Howard of New York, late assistant Surgeon U. S. A.

This Ambulance is a light, two-horse, four-wheeled carriage, designed to carry four persons besides the driver : — two recumbent, — two sitting ; or eight persons sitting.

The body of the Ambulance is mounted on elliptic springs, and the stretcher mattresses are furnished with inferior and lateral counterpoise springs, which modify or altogether prevent concussions and contribute greatly to the safety and comfort of the patients transported.

There is also connected with it a special mechanical contrivance— a "Sling" —for the suspension if necessary of wounded limbs.

Ambulances on the Howard plan were first constructed in the field before Petersburgh, Va., during the summer of 1864.

Its advantages are:—

Ist. The severely wounded are placed in, and removed from, the ambulance with but little disturbance;

2nd. Each sitting patient is well supported in a corner seat ;

3rd. Motion and shock are greatly diminished by the counterpoise springs;

4th. The Water tank is secured against injuries and leakage;

5th. A graduated litter rack ;

6th. Simplicity of construction, lightness, and strength.

2.

Nᵒ 2.   An Ambulance; known as « the Wheeling Ambulance, » *improved* by T. Morris Perot, of Philadelphia. This is a light, two-horse, four-wheeled carriage, intended to convey four persons besides the
driver : — two recumbent, —two sitting or ten persons
sitting.

Perot's improvement consists in the employment
of springs of caoutchouc,— four strong rings of this
material being secured within the body of the Ambulance and attached to levers springing from the
axletrees. It is claimed that this application secures
for the carriage an easy and agreeable movement, and
an almost entire absence of concussion, even over the
roughest roads.

Aside from Perot's improvement, the Ambulance is
in its construction similar to those which, under the
same name, were extensively employed by the U. S.
Government during the conduct of the late American
war.

3.

3.   An Ambulance; made by J. Brainard, of Boston.
This is a two-horse, four-wheeled, carriage, intended
to carry six persons besides the driver : — four recumbent,— two sitting; or ten persons sitting.

The body is mounted on « platform springs. » The mattresses and seats are arranged on what is known as the « Rucker » plan — the backs of the seats being hinged at the top, so as when opened inward and locked, to form an upper tier of mattresses.

The Ambulance exibited was employed in the Hospital service for several months during the late war.

4.

N° 4.   An Ambulance; one of thirty, of similar construction, given by citizens of Philadelphia during the war to as many fire companies of that city, and employed in conveying sick and wounded soldiers arriving at the Baltimore station across the city, — about four miles — to the New-York station.

This ambulance service was voluntarily assumed by the Firemen, and the presence of sick soldiers and the number of Ambulances needed was signalled through the electric apparatus of the Fire Department.

In the Ambulance exhibited about three thousand soldiers were transferred from station to station.

5

5.   An ambulance, — made by Dr Thomas W Evans. This ambulance was constructed with the pur-

pose of uniting a possible capacity for four recumbent, with lightness, easiness of movement, facility of loading and unloading, and simplicity. It was however not finished until the last of August. So late as to be even *hors concours* in the competition for the special prizes offered for the best ambulance by the *Société de secours aux blessés*. Nevertheless such were its considered merits, that the jury of the *société* saw fit to award to it a second prize of 500 francs, accompanied with an expression of regret that they were unable, in view of the fixed condition of the *concours* to award to it the first prize.

This ambulance can carry ten persons seated, besides the driver and one or two attendants, or four lying down and two seated, besides the driver and attendants. The seats can be used, each as a mattress, upon the floor of the wagon, the iron wheels with which they are furnished, resting when in position upon springs beneath the floor — the object was to place these supplementary springs first out of the way, secondly, where, when once fixed, they would' be secured against accidents. For the upper tier, four rings of caoutchouc are attached, in front and rear, to the sides of the wagon, 2 feet 9 inches from the floor, two rings to an upright in the centre of the wagon immediately behind the seat of the driver, and two rings to a hook which may be dropped from the rear centre. By means of this arrangement, so very

simple as scarcely to be observed unless special attention is directed to it, two ordinary French, English,
or American stretchers can be suspended *whenever*
necessary, and two additional wounded transported
inthe most confortable manner.

    This ambulance, weighing about 1,300 lbs, is
slightly heavier than the other American ambulances.
The forward wheels turn readily *under* the body of
the wagon. The top is covered with enameled cloth ;
and folding seats are placed at the rear end, outside,
for one or two attendants. It is furnished with a
double tank for ice and water, and with a box for a
few necessary supplies. Two stretchers are carried
overhead inside, and a supplementary one outside.

                        6.

Nᵒ 6.   A model of a Railway Ambulance, or « Hospital
      Car, » made by Messrs. Cummings and Son, Jersey
      City, from specifications furnished by Dr. Elisha Har-
      ris of New-York. This model is a *fac-simile* of the
      Hospital Cars employed during the war by the U. S.
      Sanitary Commission on the railway between Wa-
      shington and New-York, as well as on several other
      military railways in other portions of the United
      States.
          The model, constructed on a scale of 1/4, shows
      in detail every thing, — couches, dispensary, wine

closet, water closet, systems of ventilation and heating, etc.,—employed in the construction and equip-
ment of the Sanitary Commission Cars; while at
the same time externally it perfectly represents
the construction of an ordinary American passenger
car.

To it is attached a patent safety break, as well as a
set of self-acting ventilators, furnished by W. Crea-
mer, of New-York.

7.

N° 7.   A Horse Litter; made by F. P. Woodcock, of New-
York. This litter, for one horse or mule, is designed
to carry either one or two wounded men. If necessary
the *brancard* can readily be removed, and the saddle
and straps employed to secure the transportation of
forage or other material. The litter is light, strong,
and simple.

8.

8.   A set of Hand Litters; folding; —a form extensively
used by the U. S. Ambulance service.

9.

9.   A set of Hand Litters constructed by Dr. B. Howard
of New-York. In these litters the canvass is secured to
the shafts by loops. The design is to obviate the sometimes cruel necessity of lifting the patient from the
litter; as, by detaching the sacking, it can be readily

slipped out from beneath the patient, after he has been placed upon his mattress.

10.

N° 10.   A Hand Litter; made by S. S. Stevens and Sons, of Baltimore.

GROUP SECOND. — Ambulances of Supply.

1.

11.   A Medicine Wagon; known as Autenrieth's, — the fixtures having been furnished by G. Autenrieth, of New-York. The wagon is intended to carry for field service a full complement of the medicines authorised by the " supply table" of the Medical Bureau, also a set of Hand Litters, as well as a light compact Amputating table. Wagons of this construction were favourably regarded and most extensively employed by the U. S. Government during the late war.

2.

12.   A Medicine Wagon; known as Perot's,— constructed by T. Morris Perot, of Philadelphia. In this wagon the drawers and compartments are adapted to the carriage of medicines in bulk, in parcels, and in bottles; the system of packing being such as to secure the latter against fracture in certain instances by the employment of springs; in certain cases by the em-

ployment of columns of compressible air, obtained by a simple device.

The rear of the wagon is so constructed as to shelter the surgeon, while dispensing in the field, from rain and wind. A set of Hand Litters is carried, as also a strong Amputating table.

This wagon is a little lighter than the Autenrieth wagon, and was usually drawn by four horses.

Wagons constructed by Mr. Perot were used to a considerable extent by the U. S. Medical Bureau during the late war.

3.

Nº 15.   An Ambulance Kitchen; invented by Mr. Pinner, of New-York.

The special purpose of this Kitchen is to furnish soldiers, — particularly the sick and wounded, while on the march or on the battle field, — with hot coffee, soup, and cooked food of various kinds; while possessing all the necessary apparatus of a well-organized Kitchen, it can be used with great advantage at all temporary encampments and Hospital stations.

It is so made and furnished as to be used, — if needed, — as an Ambulance of transport.

4.

14.   A Coffee Wagon ; invented by J. Dunton, of Philadelphia. The wagon exhibited, — designed to furnish

the soldier on the march and on the field of battle with
hot coffee and tea, — was one of several in the service
of the U. S. Christian commission during the last
months of the war, and was actually employed by that
Commission,—furnishing hot coffee to the wounded of
both armies,—on the day of the surrender of Gen.
Lee, at Appomatox Court-house.

5.

Nº 15.   A Field Medicine Pannier Basket, furnished, —
made by T. Morris Perot, of Philadelphia.

6.

16.   A Medicine Pannier, furnished,— made by Jacob
Dunton, of Philadelphia.

The bottles in this Pannier are of block tin,—internal and external surfaces of tin, between which is placed a thin lamina of wood. The bottles are light and
strong, well secured at the mouth, and, as was generally the case when economy of space was desired, —
square in form.

7.

17.   Two Medicine Panniers,—made by G. Autenrieth
of New-York. These Panniers, as well as Nos. 5 et 6,
were extensively employed by the U. S. Medical
Bureau.

8.

18.   A Hospital Knapsack, — furnished, made by J.

Dunton, of Philadelphia. It is intended that this Knapsack should be carried in the field by a steward, with a suitable provision of medicines, stimulants, dressings, etc. The Knapsack is so constructed as to rest to a considerable extent on the small of the back and hips, and by its weight rather assists than otherwise the soldier in maintaining an erect position.

9.

Nº 19.   A Hospital Knapsack, furnished, — made by T. Morris Perot, of Philadelphia. It is designed to serve the same purpose as the hospital Knapsack already described.

10.

20.   A U. S. A. Pack Saddle; old pattern.

11.

21.   A U. S. A. Pack Saddle; new pattern.

CLASS II. — HOSPITALS.

GROUP FIRST. — Models and Plans.

1.

22.   A Block Model, — of the U. S. General Hospital at West Philadelphia, giving a general view of the grounds pavilions, kitchens, etc., connected with that hospital.

14

2.

Nº 23.   A Diagram,—of ground plan of the same hospital.

3.

24.   A Lithographic View,— of the same Hospital.

4.

25.   A Block Model,— of the U. S. General Hospital at Chesnut-Hill, Philadelphia, giving a general view of the grounds, pavilions, corridors, kitchens, railways, drains, etc., connected with that Hospital.

5.

26.   A Lithographic View, — of the same hospital.

6.

27.   Model of a Pavilon, — of the U. S. General Hospital at Chestnut-hill, scale, 1/24. This model shows, in *fac-simile*, the exterior and interior construction of a ward pavilon, the mode of ventilation and heating (Leed's system), the latrines, bath-rooms, and offices, together with the arrangement of beds, furniture, etc.

7.

28.   A Model, *fac-simile*, of the log-houses employed in the construction of the U. S. General Hospital at City Point, Va.; made by Capt. Isaac Harris, Brooklyn, New-York.

8.

N° 29.   A Lithograph, giving exterior and general appearance of the U. S. hospital steamer *Elm-City*.

GROUP SECOND. — Hospital Tents.

1.

50.   A Field Hospital Tent; square.— Sample of those generally issued by the U. S. Government during the war.

2.

31.   A Field Hospital Tent, called "the Umbrella-tent," made by Wm. Richardson, of Philadelphia. It is claimed that this tent occupies less space when packed, is more readily unpacked and erected, and when erected is more convenient and secure, than either the square (wall), or Sibley tents, which have hitherto been regarded with most favour.

GROUP THIRD. — Hospital Furniture.
(WITHIN TENT N° 30).

1.

32.   Eight Hospital Beds, *furnished*,—viz., 8 iron bedsteads; two patterns. 7 bedsacks, 1 water bed, 8 pillows, 8 pillow slips, 16 sheets, 8 blankets, 8 counterpanes, 8 mosquitoe bars.

2.

Nᵒ 33.   A Head-rest; made by S. S. Stevens, Baltimore.

3.

34.   A Bed-table; made by S. S. Stevens, Baltimore.

4.

35.   Camp stools.

5.

36.   Camp tables.

6.

37.   A Hospital Mess Chest; made by T. Morris Perot, of Philadelphia, — containing; — 6 tin cups, 1 tin dipper, 1 pepper box, 1 salt box, 1 grater, 6 knives and forks, 1 meat fork, 1 basin, 1 bowl, 6 iron tea spoons, 6 iron table spoons, 1 fry pan, 1 oval teapot, 1 iron tea kettle, 1 stew pan, 1 oval boiler, 6 round tin pans, 6 tin tumblers, 1 coffee boiler, 3 tin boxes for coffee, tea, and sugar.

CLASS III. — SURGICAL INSTRUMENTS AND APPARATUS

1.

58.   Staff Surgeons' capital Operating Set; containing, two amputating knives, 2 catlings, 4 scalpels, 1 cartilage knife, 1 bow saw, 2 blades, 1 metacarpal saw,

1 Hay's saw, 1 conical trephine, 1 small crown trephine, 1 Liston's bone forceps, 1 Liston's bone forceps, curved, 1 rongeur, 1 sequestrum forceps, 1 artery forceps, 12 surgeon's needles, 1 tourniquet, 1 chain saw, 1 tenaculum, 1 scissors, 1 chisel, 1 gouge, 1 mallet, 4 drills and handle, 2 retractors, 1 raspitor, 1 elevator, 1 brush, 12 yards iron wire, ⅛ oz. silk ligature, ⅛ oz. wax.

2.

N° 39. Regimental Surgeons' Field Set; containing — 2 amputating knives, 2 catlings, 5 scalpels, 2 bistouris, 1 hernia knife, 1 finger knife, 1 bow-saw, — 2 blades, 1 matacarpal saw, 1 Hay's saw, 1 conical trephine, 1 Liston's broad edged bone forceps, 1 sequestrum forceps, 1 artery forceps, 1 ball forceps, 1 dressing forceps, 1 dissecting forceps, 1 set of Mott's needles, 1 tourniquet, 1 tenaculum, 2 scissors, 2 retractors, 1 trocar and canula, 1 elevator, 1 raspitor, 1 director, 6 bougies, — silver plated, 3 silver catheters, 6 gum elastic catheters, 12 yards iron suture wire, ¼ oz. silk ligature, ⅛ oz. wax, 12 surgeons' needles.

3.

40. Staff Surgeons' Minor Operating Set; containing, — 1 amputating knife, 3 scalpels, 4 bistouris, 1 artery forceps, 1 ball forceps, 1 Galle's forceps, 1 dressing forceps, 1 dissecting forceps, 1 artery needle,

12 surgeons' needles, 1 tenaculum, 2 scissors, 1 trocar and canula, 1 Belloqnes canula, 1 bullet probe, 1 director, 6 silver-plated bougies, 3 silver catheters, 6 gum elastic catheters, 12 yards iron wire, ¼ oz. silk ligature, ⅛ oz. wax.

4.

N° 41.   Staff Surgeons' Pocket Set; containing—1 scalpel, 8 bistouris, 1 tenaculum, 1 gum lancet, 2 thumb lancets, 1 small razor, 1 artery forceps, 1 dressing forceps, 1 artery needle, 12 surgeons' needles, 1 exploring needle, 1 tenaculum needle, 1 scissors, 1 director, 3 probes, 1 caustic-holder, 1 male and female catheters, 6 yards iron wire ⅛ oz. silk suture, ⅛ oz. wax.

5.

42.   Hospital Pocket Set; containing — 1 sharp pointed bistouri, 1 probe pointed bistourie, 1 scalpel, 1 tenaculum, 1 abcess lancet, 1 compound catheter, 1 pair scissors-straight, 1 pair scissors-angular, 1 dressing forceps, 1 artery forceps, 1 spatula, 1 director, 2 probes, 6 needles, ligature, silk, wax, etc.

These five sets of surgical instruments, made by George Tiemann and Co., New York, were issued during the war by the U. S. Government in large quantities to the surgical officers of the army.

6.

43.   A case of Surgical Instruments; a Field Set, —
made by D. W. Kolbe, of Philadelphia.

The packing of this set is alone peculiar, the common rose-wood case being dispensed with.

7

44.   A case of Instruments, made by George Tiemann
and Co., showing some of the most recent improvements in American surgical mechanics, viz., *Tray
Nº 1.*—1 Simonowsky's saw, 1 parallel knife, 1 hard
rub endoscope, 1 Scattergood's passary, 1 Thomas
perforator, 1 Tiemann and Co.'s throat and bullet
forceps, 1 Emmett's improved uterine adjuster. —
Tray Nº 2.—1. Hammond's electroceps, 1 Stearn's
dilator, 1, uterine hypod syr carrier, 1 Thiebaud's
stricture dilator, 1 Edwards caustic carrier, 1 Burge's
throat forceps, 1 Tiemann's elastic bullet forceps, 1
White's hysteratome, 1 Peter's stricture cutter, 1
Elliott's uterine sound, 1 Tiemann and Co.'s bullet
forceps. — *Tray Nº 5.* — 1 Tiemann and Co.'s ton-
silatome, 1 uvula scissors and clamps, 1 uvula guil-
lotine, 1 hard rubber and drill'd steel cork for champagne bottle, 1 Chisolm's chloroform inhaler, 2 rub
pill bougies, 1 sponge carrier for finger, 1 Church's
tongue depresser, 1 Ellsburg's do., do., 1 Carrol's
knot tightener, 1 Stock's eylid compresser, 1 Noyes

irridictomy scissors, 1 Tiemann and Co.'s entrapia
tome and forceps, 1 fenestra and artery forceps, 1
entrap and forceps (Morton's), 1 Fisher's phymosis
forceps and screw, 1 Sand's needle forceps, 1 Richardson's sponge holder, Thomas and Co.'s irridictomy and ptrigion forceps, 1 Altrap's forceps. —
Tray N° 4.—1 Phair's 3-bladed speculum, 1 Thomas'
new ditto, Emmett's ditto, 1 Tiemann and Co.'s 5
valve ditto, 1 Thomas and Co.'s 4 valve ditto, 1 Sims'
rectum dilator. — *Tray N °5.* —1 handle, 1 amputating saw, 2 knives, 1 handle and 7 pocket instruments (Tieman's patent).

8.

45.   A set of Splints, made by A. M. Day, of Benning-
ton Vt., viz., extension bar and gaiter, 1 large double
inclined plane, 1 medium double inclined plane, 1
small double inclined plane, 8 radius splints, 6 fore
arm, 5 inter-osseous, 5 joint arm, 5 condyle and
humerus, 2 clavicle, 5 dressing splints, 4 patella
splints, 12 ankle splints.

9.

46.   A Set of Splints, made by the " Surgical Splint
Co." Winsted. C'.

10.

47.   Perforated zinc Splint and Shears ; furnished by the
U. S. Sanitary Commission.

11.

Nᵒ 48   A Fracture Apparatus, made by Dr. Gurdon Buck, of New-York, accompanied with a bed and manikin, showing the mode of applying the same.

12.

49.   A Fracture Bed; invented by Dr. M. M. Latta of Goshen, Indiana.

13.

50.   An Apparatus, for fractures of the inferior maxillary, made by Dr. C. S. Bean, of Baltimore.

14.

51.   An Invalid Bed, invented by Dr. Josiah Crosby, of Manchester, N. H. The design is to secure a change of linen and a fulfilment of certain natural offices without a change of position on the part of the patient. Many of these beds were used in the U. S. General Hospitals.

15.

52.   An Invalid Elevator; made by Mr. Marx, of New York.   Design similar to that of the Invalid Bed.

16.

53.   A set of Artificial Limbs, for amputations of the fore arm, arm, thigh, and foot, together with Appa-

ratus for ex-sections at the elbow and shoulder joints ;
made by Dr. Hudson, of New York·

17.

54. An Artificial Leg ; made by D. W. Kolbe, of Philadelphia.

18.

55. An Instrument for the better anæsthetic administration of sulphuric ether, invented by Dr. F. D.
Lente, Cold Springs, N. Y.

19.

56. An Apparatus, for the production and administration of nitrous oxide gas, with the view of thereby
inducing anæsthesia, — prepared by Dr. J. Q. Colton,
of New York, who claims that he has first successfully
demonstrated the anæsthetic properties of the nitrous
oxide gas, and the special advantages of its employment in a large class of cases, as a substitute for
chloroform and ether.

20.

57. A Preparation illustrating a method of operating
in cases of compound fracture, — prepared by Dr. B.
Howard, of New York.

CLASS IV. -- SANITARY SUPPLIES.

GROUP FIRST. — Clothing.

SAMPLES OF THAT USED BY THE U. S. SANITARY COMMISSION.

I.

N° 58. Blankets, and Bed quilts.

2.

59. Bed sacks.

3.

60 Cushions.

4.

61. Drawers.

5.

62. Handkerchiefs.

6.

63. Mittens.

7.

64. Sheets.

8.

65. Shirts and dressing-gowns.

9.

66. Socks (cotton and woollen), and slippers

10.

67. Towels.

GROUP SECOND. — Food.

SAMPLES OF THAT USED BY THE U. S. SANITARY COMMISSION.

1.

Nº 68.   Apple butter.

2.

69.   Barley.

3.

70.   Beef, dried.

4.

71.   Beef stock (Martinez).

5.

72.   Broma (Baker's).

6.

73.   Cabbage, pickled.

7.

74.   Canned fruits.

8.

75.   Canned meats.

9.

76.   Canned vegetables.

10.

77.   Catsup.

11.

78.   Cheese.

12.

N° 79.   Chocolate (Baker's).

13.

80.   Cocoa (Baker's).

14.

81.   Codfish.

15.

82.   Coffee-extract (Borden's).

16.

83.   Condensed Milk (Borden's).

17.

84.   Corn, dried, sweet.

18.

85.   Corn, pop.

19.

86.   Crackers and biscuit.

20.

87.   Dried fruits.

21.

88.   Eggs, desiccated (Lamont's).

22.

89.   Extracts, flavoring (Woodruff's).

23.

90.   Farina (Hecker's).

24.

Nº 91.   Flax seed.

25.

92.   Groats.

26.

93.   Hickory nuts.

27.

94.   Hominy.

28.

95.   Iceland Moss.

29.

96.   Jellies.

30.

97.   Julienne soup.

31.

98.   Lemonade condensed (Morris').

32.

99.   Lemon extract.

33.

100.   Lemon syrup.

34.

101.   Lemons.

35.

102.   Lime juice.

36.

103.   Maccaroni.

37.

N° 104.   Maizena.

38.

105.   Molasses.

39.

106.   Mustard.

40.

107.   Nutmegs.

41.

108.   Oatmeal.

42.

109.   Oranges.

43.

110.   Oysters, pickled.

44.

111.   Pickles.

45.

112.   Potatoes.

46.

113.   Prunes.

47.

114.   Rice.

48.

115.   Sago.

49.

116.   Sardines.

50.

Nº 117.   Spices, assorted.

51.

118.   Sugar b. and w.

52.

119.   Tapioca.

53.

120.   Tea b. and g.

54.

121.   Tobacco (Messrs. Gail and Ax, Baltimore, and Dumont, New-York).

55.

122.   Vegetables, desiccated.

56.

123.   Vermicelli.

57.

124.   Yeast powder.

58.

125.   Ale, pale (Mc Pherson and Donald Smith, New-York).

59.

126.   Blackberry brandy.

60.

127.   Brandy (F. S. Cozzens, New-York).

61.

Nº 128.   Cider, Champagne (J. Kierman, New-York).

62.

129.   Extract of Jam. Ginger, (Fred. Brown.)

63.

130.   Rum, Jamaica (F. S. Cozzens.)

64.

131.   Raspberry vinegar.

65.

132.   Syrups.

66.

133.   Whiskey;two Star, Old Rye, Bourbon, (F. S. Cozzens.)

67.

154.   Domestic Wines; F. S. Cozzens, viz. Los Angelos Madeira, Los Angelos Sherry, Native Claret, Pride of Sandusky, Cabinet Catawba, Dry Catawba, Empire P. B. sparkling Catawba.

68.

135.   Foreign wines : Port, sherry, etc., F. S. Cozzens.

15

1.

Nº 136.   A Sanitary Commission Tool Case, containing—a large axe, 2 hatchets, 3 hammers, 2 saws, 1 auger, 2 wrenches, half a dozen gimlets, 1 sardine opener, 1 corkscrew, 1 pocket corkscrew, 1 ice pick, 1 spring punch, 1 farrier knife, 1 butcher knife, 1 drawing knife, 1 pair shears, 1 polished steel box opener, 1 pot brace, 1 Jennings bit, 2 chisels, 1 firmer chisel, 1 Ames spade, nails and rivets.

2.

137.   A Sanitary Commission Mess Kit, viz. ;—a nest of camp kettles, 5 mess pans, 1 Dutch oven, $\frac{1}{2}$ dozen knives and forks, $\frac{1}{2}$ dozen table spoons (iron), $\frac{1}{2}$ dozen tea spoons (iron), cups, dippers, tin basins, tin plates, a wine cooler, a water cooler, knives and forks.

3.

138.   An Officer's Mess Chest ; — T. Morris Perot, Philadelphia ; containing, 1 camp stove, 1 oven, 2 mess-pans, 1 boiler, 1 mess kettle, 1 sauce pan, 1 teapot, 1 coffee pot, 1 knife case, 12 knives and forks, 1 spooncase, 6 tea spoons, 6 table-spoons, 6 tumblers, 6 cups, 1 frying pan, 1 gridiron, 1 tin-tray, 2 tin dishes, 1 tea kettle, 1 pepperbox, 1 saltbox,

6 tin basins, 2 washhand basins, 6 plates, 1 dipper, 1 ladle, 1 grater, 4 boxes for butter, tea, coffee, sugar, 4 mugs.

4.

139.   A Field Mess Chest; T. Morris Perot, Philadelphia, containing — 2 large iron boilers, 5 camp kettles, 1 knife case with 2 dozen knives and forks, 1 spoon case with 1 dozen iron spoons, 1 meat fork, 1 dozen plates, 1 dozen cups, 5 dippers, 1 gridiron, 1 salt-box, 1 pepper-box.

5.

140.   A Mess Pannier; J. Dunton, Philadelphia; containing — stove, coffee pot, pepper, salt, and butter box, cups, plates, knives and forks, etc.

SAMPLES USED BY THE U. S. SANITARY COMMISSION.

6.

141.   Adhesive plaster.

7.

142.   Alcohol.

8.

143.   Bandages.

9.

Baskets.

10.

Brooms.

11.

Nº 146. Brushes.

12.

147. Buckets.

13.

148. Buttons.

14.

149. Candlesticks.

15.

150. Combs.

16.

151. Chairs.

17.

152. Coffeepots.

18.

153. Cologne.

19.

154. Comforts.

20.

155. Cotton batting.

21.

156. Crutches.

22.

157. Envelopes for soldiers' letters.

23.

158. Eye shades.

24.

Nº 159.   Fans.

25.

160.   Feeding cups.

26.

161.   Feeding tubes.

27.

162.   Games.

28.

163.   Lanterns.

29.

164.   Letter paper (Collins Brothers.)

30.

165.   Lint.

31.

166.   Oakum.

32.

167.   Oil silk.

33.

168.   Pens and pencils for soldiers.

34.

169.   Paper bags.

35.

170.   Pins.

36.

171.   Pipes.

37.

N° 172.   Sponges.

38.

173.   Spit cups.

39.

174.   Yarn.

40.

175.   The American combined Knife and Fork ; for the use of those having but one hand.

CLASS V. — MATERIAL, HISTORICAL, AND CO-ORDINATE.

GROUP FIRST

1.

176.   Histoire de la Commission Sanitaire des États-Unis, by Dr. Thomas W. Evans.

2.

177.   Discourse of the Rev. Dr. Bellows, President of the U.S. Sanitary Commission.

3.

178.   Reply to the question " Why the Sanitary Commission need so much money, " by Mr. Knapp.

4.

Nᵒ 179.　Memorial of the Great Central fair held in behalf
of the U. S. Sanitary Commission, by Mr. C. J. Stillé.

5.

180.　Military Statistics of the United States, by Mr.
Elliot.

. 6.

181.　Tribute book, by Mr. Goodrich.

7.

182.　Essais sur la chirurgie et la médecine militaire

8.

183.　Three weeks at Gettysburg.

9.

184.　A brief history of the operations of the U. S. Sanitary Commission.

10.

185.　History of the U. S. Sanitary Commission.

11.

186.　Essais d'hygiène et de thérapeutique militaire, by
Dr. Thomas. W. Evans.

12.

187.　Les Institutions sanitaires pendant le conflit Aus-
tro-Prussien, by Dr. Thomas W. Evans.

13.

Nº 188.   Military medical and surgical essays, edited by
Dr. Hammond.

14.

189   Charts, Diagrams, etc., of the U. S. Sanitary
Commission.

15.

190.   Photographs of places made memorable by the
war.

16.

191.   Guerre d'Amérique.

17.

192.   Model Libraries, furnished Camps and Hospitals,
by the U. S. Christian Commission.

18.

193.   Five groups in terre cuite, by Rogers.

19.

194.   Lithograph of the bazaar of the Sanitary Commission at Philadelphia.

20.

195.   Photograph of Pinner's kitchen ambulance.

21.

196.   Tickets given by the Christian Commission to each

soldier bearing his name, age, number of regiment, etc.

22.

N° 197. A roll containing the autographs of 19,108 persons who have undergone surgical operations without pain while under the influence of nitrous oxyde gas, administered by Dr. J. Q. Colton.

23.

198. Plan of the Chestnut Hill Hospital at Philadelphia.

24.

199. Picture frame made by a wounded soldier.

25.

200. The wounded soldier.

26.

201. Tribute from Dusseldorf artists to the ladies of New York.

27.

202. Frame enclosing various photographs, medals, etc., of the U. S. Sanitary Commission.

28.

203. De la découverte du caoutchouc vulcanisé et de la priorité de son application à la chirurgie civile et militaire. Brochure, by Dr. Thomas W Evans.

29.

204   Treatise on military surgery, Hamilton.

30.

205.   Army Regulations (U. S.)

31.

206.   Various publications of or pertaining to the U. S. Sanitary Commission.

32.

207.   Ambulance and sanitary material, by Dr Thomas W. Evans.

33.

208.   Dentistry and the material it employs, by Dr Thomas W. Evans.

34.

209.   Platform scales.

35.

210.   Balances.

36.

211.   Anthropomètre.

37.

212.   Spiromètre.

N°s 32, 33, 34, 35. — (Instruments used by Inspectors of the Sanitary Commission while conducting observations to determine the weight, strength, physical developement, etc., of soldiers recruited in different sections of the country, or representing different elements of population or social condition.)

38.

Nº 213.   A Sanitary Commission mail-bag of the Army of the Potomac.

39.

214.   Flags of the U. S. Sanitary Commission.

40.

215.   Rubber loops; used in one of the U. S. Sanitary Commission Hospital cars.

41.

216.   A Rebel canteen.

GROUP SECOND.

1.

217.   An "Umbrella tent; " Officer's, — made by Wm. Richardson, Philadelphia, constructed as No. 30.

2.

218.   An " Umbrella tent, " Officer's; — height 11 feet, diameter at base 13 1/2, form octagonal, supported by a telescopic centre pole, slender T iron rafters, and eight light wooden props.

The same advantages are claimed as for No. 30; maker, N. Walton, of Saint-Louis.

3.

Nº 219. A Hospital Tent; square (wall), similar to No. 50,

4.

220. A Lifeboat; made of gutta percha.

5.

221. A model of a California stove; illustrating a mode of heating tents, employed in the American Army.

The system was generally regarded by medical officers as particularly adapted to the heating of Hospital tents, where a uniform temperature was especially desired.

6.

222. Samples of clothing issued by the United States Government during the war to infantry soldiers, namely, overcoat, coat, trowsers, shoes, stockings, shirt, drawers, cap, etc.

7.

223. Spike candlestick.

8.

224. Combined splint and fracture bed, Dr. J. Langer.

9.

225. Bed and pillow for the sick or wounded, Madame Petiteau.

CONTENTS

CHAPTER FIRST. — The Sanitary Commission of the United States and the convention of Geneva. — Disposition of modern nations to mitigate sufferings occasioned by war. — Sanitary Commission of the United States. — Initiative of American women. — Conferences of Geneva. — Principles of the Geneva convention analogous to those expressed in the statutes of American Sanitary Commission. — Establishment of international Relief Societies favored by several sovereigns.   1

CHAPTER II. — Origin of the Prussian Society of relief for the wounded. — Sympathy of the King and Queen of Prussia for the work of the Sanitary Commission of the United States. — Autograph letter from the King. — Groups of voluntary hospital attendants at the different railway stations. — First appearance of the Prussian Relief Society. — Its activity during the Schleswig-Holstein compaign. — Sending of commissioners to Schleswig   . .   .   17

CHAPTER III. — Transformation of the Central Society into an international Relief Society. — Resources of War Departement, however considerable, are generally insufficient. — Necessity of spontaneous action on the part of populations. — The Prussian Society of relief to the sick and wounded obtains the privilege of corporation. — Appeal of the central committee to the nation. — Central depot of Berlin. — Reflections suggested by it to the author. — Statutes of the Prussian Relief Society.   .   29

CHAPTER IV. — Combat of Langensalza. — Obstinacy of the struggle. — The town of Langensalza encumbered with wounded. — Complete insufficiency of resources in the medical service of the Hanovrian army and the Prussian detachment. — Distress of the surgeons. — Their joy at the sight of the relief sent forward by the central committee of Berlin.   51

CHAPTER V. — The battle of Sadowa.— Magnitude of the struggle. Heart-rending scenes. — Large number of wounded remain several days without dressing of wounds. — Activity and devotedness of Prussian physicians. — Hospitals in the villages surrounding the battle field. — Solicitude and kindness of the surgeons in the field hospitals. — The wounded in the hospitals of Milowitz and Sadowa.   59

CHAPTER VI. — Activity of the Prussian Society. — Important convoys shipped to the theatre of war. — Depots established in Bohemia and on the banks of the Mein. — International character of the Prussian Relief Society. — Buffets established in the stations of the railways to distribute refreshments to the troops. — Prussian Society distributes books. — Disinterestedness and devotedness of the agents of the Society. — The journal Krieger-heil.   75

CHAPTER VII. — Knights of the orders of Saint John and Malta.— Services rendered by these orders during the war. — Hospitals of Berlin. Activity of the Queen and Princess Royal of Prussia in favor of the relief societies.   95

CHAPTER VIII. — Relief Societies in Saxony and southern Germany. — The Saxon Relief Society. — General de Reitzenstein. — Sanitary Society of Wurtemberg. — Elevated views of the Queen of Wurtembourg upon the mission of sanitary institutions. — The Badischer Frauenverein. — Zeal and devotion of the Grand-Duchess and Princess Wilhelm. — Sanitary movement in Bavaria.   107

CHAPTER IX. — Austrian Relief Societies. — The Patriotischer Damenverein — Princess de Schwarzenberg places her palace at the disposition of the ladies association. — Devotion of madame de Lowenthal. — The Patriotic Society renders great services to the army. — The Holzhospital. — Heroic conduct of two women.   125

CHAPTER X. — The Italian Society of relief to the wounded. — Medical Society of Milan, under the impulsion of its president, organizes the first local Relief Society. — Appeal of this association to Italy. — Committee of the Milanese Society recognized as central committee of the Italian Society of Relief to the wounded. At the time of war the Florentine committee establishes itself as central committee of the societies situated south of the Pô. — Discussions following this incident. — Services rendered by the Italian Society of relief to the wounded 155

CHAPTER XI. — Conclusion. — Relief Societies in operation during the last war have not offered any marked progress or improvment upon the proceedings employed by the United States Sanitary commission. — Utility of sanitary collections. — The author's American sanitary collection. — Russia's adhesion to the Geneva convention. — International exhibition of Societies of Relief for the wounded. — Happy results of this exhibition. 147

Appendix. — Essay on ambulance wagons. . 167

Universal exhibition — rewards and letters.. . . . 183

Catalogue of articles forming the United States sanitary collection of Dr Thomas W. Evans 197

PARIS. — PRINTED BY SIMON RAÇON AND Cᵉ, I, ERFURTH STREET.

www.ingramcontent.com/pod-product-compliance
Lightning Source LLC
Chambersburg PA
CBHW030402270326
41926CB00009B/1223